BIOLOGY AND THERAPY OF ACUTE LEUKEMIA

DEVELOPMENTS IN ONCOLOGY

F.J. Cleton and J.W.I.M. Simons, eds.: Genetic Origins of Tumour Cells. 90-247-2272-1.
J. Aisner and P. Chang, eds.: Cancer Treatment and Research. 90-247-2358-2.
B.W. Ongerboer de Visser, D.A. Bosch and W.M.H. van Woerkom-Eykenboom, eds.: Neuro-oncology: Clinical and Experimental Aspects. 90-247-2421-X.
K. Hellmann, P. Hilgard and S. Eccles, eds.: Metastasis: Clinical and Experimental Aspects. 90-247-2424-4.
H.F. Seigler, ed.: Clinical Management of Melanoma. 90-247-2584-4.
P. Correa and W. Haenszel, eds.: Epidemiology of Cancer of the Digestive Tract. 90-247-2601-8.
L.A. Liotta and I.R. Hart, eds.: Tumour Invasion and Metastasis. 90-247-2611-5.
J. Banoczy, ed.: Oral Leukoplakia. 90-247-2655-7.
C. Tijssen, M. Halprin and L. Endtz, eds.: Familial Brain Tumours. 90-247-2691-3.
F.M. Muggia, C.W. Young and S.K. Carter, eds.: Anthracycline Antibiotics in Cancer. 90-247-2711-1.
B.W. Hancock, ed.: Assessment of Tumour Response. 90-247-2712-X.
D.E. Peterson, ed.: Oral Complications of Cancer Chemotherapy. 0-89838-563-6.
R. Mastrangelo, D.G. Poplack and R. Riccardi, eds.: Central Nervous System Leukemia. Prevention and Treatment. 0-89838-570-9.
A. Polliack ed.: Human Leukemias. Cytochemical and Ultrastructural Techniques in Diagnosis and Research. 0-89838-585-7.
W. Davis, C. Maltoni and S. Tanneberger, eds.: The Control of Tumor Growth and its Biological Bases. 0-89838-603-9.
A.P.M. Heintz, C. Th. Griffiths and J.B. Trimbos, eds.: Surgery in Gynecological Oncology. 0-89838-604-7.
M.P. Hacker, E.B. Double and I. Krakoff, eds.: Platinum Coordination Complexes in Cancer Chemotherapy. 0-89838-619-5.
M.J. van Zwieten. The Rat as Animal Model in Breast Cancer Research: A Histopathological Study of Radiation- and Hormone-Induced Rat Mammary Tumors. 0-89838-624-1.
B. Löwenberg and A. Hogenbeck, eds.: Minimal Residual Disease in Acute Leukemia. 0-89838-630-6.
I. van der Waal and G.B. Snow, eds.: Oral Oncology. 0-89838-631-4.
B.W. Hancock and A.M. Ward, eds.: Immunological Aspects of Cancer. 0-89838-664-0.
K.V. Honn and B.F. Sloane, eds.: Hemostatic Mechanisms and Metastasis. 0-89838-667-5.
K.R. Harrap, W. Davis and A.N. Calvert, eds.: Cancer Chemotherapy and Selective Drug Development. 0-89838-673-X.
V.D. Velde, J.H. Cornelis and P.H. Sugarbaker, eds.: Liver Metastasis. 0-89838-648-5.
D.J. Ruiter, K. Welvaart and S. Ferrone, eds.: Cutaneous Melanoma and Precursor Lesions. 0-89838-689-6.
S.B. Howell, ed.: Intra-Arterial and Intracavitary Cancer Chemotherapy. 0-89838-691-8.
D.L. Kisner and J.F. Smyth, eds.: Interferon Alpha-2: Pre-Clinical and Clinical Evaluation. 0-89838-701-9.
P. Furmanski, J.C. Hager and M.A. Rich, eds.: RNA Tumor Viruses, Oncogenes, Human Cancer and Aids: On the Frontiers of Understanding. 0-89838-703-5.
J.E. Talmadge, I.J. Fidler and R.K. Oldham: Screening for Biological Response Modifiers: Methods and Rationale. 0-89838-712-4.
J.C. Bottino, R.W. Opfell and F.M. Muggia, eds.: Liver Cancer. 0-89838-713-2.
P.K. Pattengale, R.J. Lukes and C.R. Taylor, eds.: Lymphoproliferative Diseases: Pathogenesis, Diagnosis, Therapy. 0-89838-725-6.
F. Cavalli, G. Bonadonna and M. Rozencweig, eds.: Malignant Lymphomas and Hodgkin's Disease. 0-89838-727-2.

BIOLOGY AND THERAPY OF ACUTE LEUKEMIA

Proceedings of the
Seventeenth Annual Detroit Cancer Symposium
Detroit, Michigan — April 12-13, 1984

edited by

Laurence Baker
Frederick Valeriote
Voravit Ratanatharathorn

Wayne State University
Detroit, Michigan

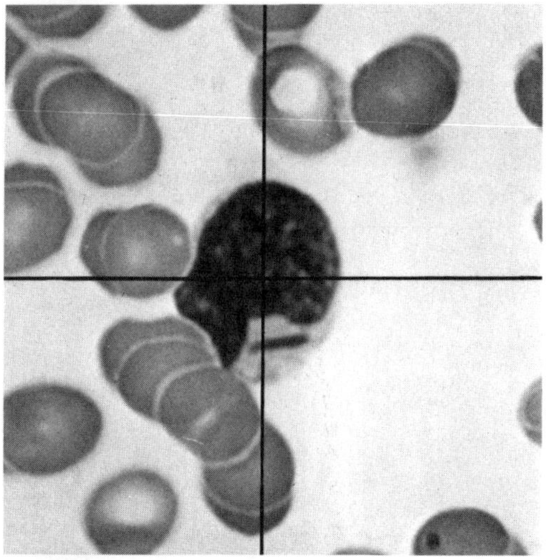

Martinus Nijhoff Publishing
a member of the Kluwer Academic Publishers Group
Boston/Dordrecht/Lancaster

Distributors for North America:
Kluwer Academic Publishers
190 Old Derby Street
Hingham, MA 02043

Distributors for all other countries:
Kluwer Academic Publishers Group
Distribution Centre
P.O. Box 322
3300 AH Dordrecht
The Netherlands

This Symposium was presented by Wayne State University School of Medicine, Division of Oncology; Comprehensive Cancer Center of Metropolitan Detroit; and Harper-Grace Hospitals.

Editorial Assistant: Ms. Linda Leino

Library of Congress Cataloging in Publication Data

Detroit Cancer Symposium (17th : 1984)
Biology and therapy of acute leukemia.

(Developments in oncology)
1. Leukemia—Congresses. 2. Leukemia—Treatment—Congresses. I. Baker, Laurence H. II. Valeriote, Frederick. III. Ratanatharathorn, Voravit. IV. Title. V. Series. [DNLM: 1. Leukemia—congresses. 2. Leukemia—therapy—congresses. W1 DE998N / WH 250 D483 1984b]
RC643.D47 1984 616.99'419 85-7092
ISBN 0-89838-728-0

Printed in the United States of America

CONTENTS

LIST OF PARTICIPANTS

Frederick R. Appelbaum, M.D.
Associate Professor of Medicine
University of Washington School of Medicine
Associate Member, Fred Hutchinson
Cancer Research Center
Seattle, Washington

Laurence H. Baker, D.O.
Professor of Medicine
Director, Division of Medical Oncology
Department of Medicine
Wayne State University
Deputy Director of the Comprehensive
Cancer Center of Metropolitan Detroit
Detroit, Michigan

Alexander Bloch, Ph.D.
Principal Cancer Research Scientist
Department of Experimental Therapeutics
Roswell Park Memorial Institute
Buffalo, New York

James M. Boyett, Ph.D.
Statistician, Statistical Office
Pediatric Oncology Group
University of Florida
Gainesville, Florida

Irvin S.Y. Chen, Ph.D.
Assistant Professor of Medicine
Division of Hematology/Oncology
Department of Medicine
UCLA School of Medicine
Los Angeles, California

Steven J. Collins, M.D.
Assistant Professor of Medicine
University of Washington
Seattle, Washington

Kenneth A. Foon, M.D.
Head, Clinical Investigations Section
Biological Response Modifiers Program
National Cancer Institute
Frederick, Maryland

Emil J Freireich, M.D., D.Sc. (Hon.)
Chairman, Department of Hematology
The University of Texas System Cancer Center
M.D. Anderson Hospital and Tumor Institute
Houston, Texas

Judith C. Gasson, Ph.D.
Assistant Professor of Medicine
Division of Hematology/Oncology
Department of Medicine
UCLA School of Medicine
Los Angeles, California

David W. Golde, M.D.
Professor of Medicine
Chief, Division of Hematology/Oncology
Department of Medicine
UCLA School of Medicine
Los Angeles, California

David L. Hines, Ph.D.
Assistant Member
Biomedical Research Lab
Trudeau Institute, Inc.
Saranac Lake, New York

Chatchada Karanes, M.D.
Assistant Professor of Medicine
Division of Medical Oncology
Wayne State University
Detroit, Michigan

David Kessel, Ph.D.
Professor of Medicine
Division of Medical Oncology
Wayne State University
Detroit, Michigan

Father Joe Mahoney, M.Div.
Chaplain for the Bone Marrow Transplantation
and Hematologic Malignancies Service
Harper-Grace Hospitals
Detroit, Michigan

Margarita Palutke, M.D.
Professor of Pathology
Head, Section of Hematopathology,
Pathology Department
Wayne State University
Detroit, Michigan

John A. Penner, M.D.
Professor of Internal Medicine
Director, Hematology/Oncology Section
Michigan State University
East Lansing, Michigan

Harvey D. Preisler, M.D.
Deputy Chief
Department of Medical Oncology
Roswell Park Memorial Institute
Buffalo, New York

Voravit Ratanatharathorn, M.D.
Head, Bone Marrow Transplantation Unit
Department of Medicine
Division of Medical Oncology
Wayne State University
Detroit, Michigan

Yaddanapudi Ravindranath, M.B., B.S.
Associate Professor of Pediatrics
Wayne State University
Children's Hospital of Michigan
Detroit, Michigan

Michael T. Rooney, M.D.
Valley Medical Center
Lewiston, Idaho

E. Donnall Thomas, M.D.
Professor of Medicine
University of Washington School of Medicine
Associate Director for Clinical Research,
Fred Hutchinson Cancer Research Center
Seattle, Washington

Frederick A. Valeriote, Ph.D.
Professor of Medicine
Associate Director
Division of Medical Oncology
Wayne State University
Detroit, Michigan

Teresa J. Vietti, M.D.
Professor of Pediatrics
Mallinckrodt Dept. of Pediatrics
Washington University School of Medicine
Division of Hematology/Oncology
St. Louis Children's Hospital
St. Louis, Missouri

William Wachsman, M.D., Ph.D.
Fellow, Div. of Hematology/Oncology
Department of Medicine
UCLA School of Medicine
Los Angeles, California

PREFACE

This year notes two major changes in the annual Detroit Cancer Symposium. The first is our intention of selecting topics of broad interest to the cancer community and examining the subject from both a basic laboratory and clinical viewpoint. In this way, the importance of both elements of cancer research are noted and the interplay between them emphasized. Further, we believe that Symposia such as this act to stimulate the basic scientist and clinician to continue their studies with the knowledge of the impact that each has upon the other and the necessary cooperation required to solve the cancer problem. The second change is the publication of this Symposium. The previous sixteen were not committed to manuscript form. Given the change in format and intent of the series, we believe that this and subsequent volumes will make important contributions to the cancer literature.

The topic of "Biology and Therapy of Acute Leukemia" was chosen for the first Symposium because of its historical significance in cancer chemotherapy. The therapeutic rationale for human leukemia is the result of understanding the basic tumor biology largely derived from transplantable leukemias in experimental animals. It is through these models, as discussed by Dr. Fred Valeriote, that we learned the cellular kinetics of leukemia, the antileukemic effects of new agents and the effect of growth perturbation by various chemotherapeutic agents and their combinations. The influence of basic knowledge in the therapy of human leukemia is evident in the design of clinical trials over the past four decades and is demonstrated by dose-schedule oriented combination chemotherapy, re-induction chemotherapy using non-cross resistant regimens, immunotherapy and bone marrow transplantation. While it is clear that experimental models have significantly contributed to the basic formulation of current treatment strategy, we must also recognize both the limitations of these models and the biological differences between mice and humans. Consequently, we cannot expect that a single strategy would work for all patients whether the rationale is from either experimental or clinical studies. This latter point was elegantly elaborated by Dr. Emil Freireich where he has identified pronounced response heterogeneity of patients to standard therapies and is identifying these different subpopulations. Newer methods of classification of leukemic cells by cytochemistry and immunologic phenotypes described by Drs. Kenneth Foon and Margarita Palutke is perhaps one of the most obvious examples of demonstrating and analyzing tumor heterogeneity. Possibly these tools will allow us to explain the unique clinical expressions in certain subtypes of leukemia. Studies reported here from Dr. David Hine's laboratory provide an experimental demonstration of clonal variability in retrovirus transformed leukemia cells and in particular, heterogeneity in differentiation capabilities.

An important goal of this symposium was to examine and update the current therapeutic results. Complete and critical reviews of the clinical trials in acute lymphoblastic leukemia were provided by Drs. Teresa Vietti and Y. Ravindranath for childhood leukemia. Drs. Michael Rooney and Harvey Preisler carried out a parallel analysis for acute non-lymphocytic leukemia. The role of allogeneic bone marrow transplantation in acute non-lymphocytic leukemia was summarized by Dr. Fred Appelbaum, particularly the results of patients in first remission. Other new avenues of therapy such as autologous bone marrow transplantation and the use of differentiating agents were also reviewed. The difficult task of discussing the transfusion support, and management of thrombotic and hemorrhagic complications were undertaken by Drs. Chatchada Karanes and John Penner.

Prospects for the future lie in many areas. Therapeutic interventions can take account of recent basic studies in drug resistance and cell differentiation. The paramount problem of drug resistance, the varied underlying biochemical basis, as well as potential solutions to the problem were discussed by Dr. David Kessel. The intriguing possibility of controlling or modifying the differentiation "program" of a tumor cell was reviewed by Dr. Alexander Bloch. In this regard, use of potentially non-toxic differentiating factors for leukemia would be a major therapeutic advance. An exciting and topical area of research at the present time involves the role oncogenes may play in the biology, diagnosis and therapy of leukemia as exemplified in the discussions of oncogene expression. Dr. Steven Collins reviewed the specific oncogenes associated to date with experimental and human leukemias and their possible "normal" role in cellular physiology. In terms of a specific leukemia virus, the discussion of human tumor leukemia virus (HTLV) and specifically the characterization by Dr. David Golde of HTLV-II, demonstrates why a major and radical breakthrough in our understanding of the biology of leukemogenesis seems imminent.

We believe that this monograph will be valuable to basic scientists as well as clinicians who have interests in the field of acute leukemia. Reviews of the history of therapy, present-day treatment rationale and future, though now experimental, therapies are analyzed and discussed.

1

THE IMPACT OF TREATMENT ON THE NATURAL HISTORY OF ACUTE LEUKEMIA

Emil J Freireich, M.D., D.Sc. (Hon.)

The disease leukemia has been an important disease for the understanding of human malignancy. The primary reason for this is that it has been recognized almost from the time the disease was described that it is systemic from the outset and has no local presentation. As a result, it has been a prototype disease for the understanding of the biology of widespread, metastatic, systemic cancer (1). I have always felt that the clinical scientist has the opportunity to conduct basic research. Basic in the sense that it leads to a fundamental understanding of biology which almost certainly could not be observed by the laboratory scientist. Cancer, as a fundamental problem in biology, shines as an example in support of this contention. Cancer was recognized as a disease in man and further clinical study led to the appreciation that these tumors arose in organs consequently spreading regionally and ultimately systemically. These fundamental clinical observations led to the formulation of cancer biology principles which guided basic research into tumor biology for almost a century.

A second important point is that therapy as conducted by clinical scientists reveals basic biological facts about malignancy which again could not otherwise be understood or appreciated. The local-regional-systemic hypothesis of tumor biology also has guided the basic concepts of cancer treatment. This led to the important advances of surgery and radiation therapy which proved to be curative for a substantial fraction of tumor diagnoses. The enormous success of the local-regional treatment modalities reinforced the biological formulation of the natural history of cancer and led to the notion that cancer control could be accomplished exclusively by early detection and effective local treatment modalities. Prior to 1947, the possibility that systemic cancers could be cured was considered idle or quackery. However, the observation of complete hematological remissions in children with acute leukemia encouraged investigators to develop treatment strategies which have ultimately proven to be curative for approximately one half of children and at least 15% of adults with this diagnosis (2). The first systemic cancer to be cured with chemotherapy was widespread metastatic choriocarcinoma, but this tumor is unique in representing an allografted tumor derived from the fetus. It was not until the demonstration of curative treatment for acute leukemia and subsequently for Hodgkin's disease and lymphoma that it was clear that widespread systemic malignancy could be cured.

The observation that progressively improving methods of detection and progressively more radical local-regional therapies had only a slight effect in decreasing mortality from metastatic cancer; combined with the observations that leukemia, as a systemic malignancy, could be cured have led clinical scientists to now appreciate that many common forms of cancer may resemble acute leukemia and be systemic virtually from the outset. It is probably true that the continuing mortality as a result of widespread metastatic cancer results both from progression of tumors which arise locally, spread regionally and ultimately systemically and the major fraction of common malignancies which metastasize so early that they are analogous to the disease acute leukemia.

It is for these reasons that a meeting devoted to current innovative approaches to the understanding of acute leukemia holds the potential for significantly advancing our understanding of the common metastatic malignancies.

1. TREATMENT REVEALS THE HETEROGENEITY IN THE DISEASE

Once treatments are discovered which can induce complete remission in a metastatic or stage IV malignancy, such as acute leukemia, it often becomes evident that the fraction of patients who respond to a given treatment are distinctive from the fraction of patients who fail to respond to treatment. In the case of adult acute leukemia, as an example, current multiple agent combination chemotherapy can result in frequencies of complete hematological remission consistently in excess of 65%. Analysis of the subsets of patients treated with uniform combination regimens reveals that age is the single most significant variable in predicting response (3). In general, the older the patient the lower the probability of response. Detailed analysis of the meaning of the age variable in terms of response to treatment has revealed that it is made up of two components. The first relates to the overall physiological health of the host; for treatments with relatively low therapeutic indices, it is clear that ability to tolerate treatment is inversely related to age. But more important is the second component which is the frequency of type I resistance to combination chemotherapy; that is, a failure to achieve adequate cytoreduction which is also inversely related to age (4). It is for this reason that is, an association of resistant leukemia in a progressively less competent host, that age emerges as the single most important prognostic variable.

Other features which predict for outcome include objective evidence of infection, documented by fever, which is prognostically negative. The existence of other major organ failures such as liver or kidney is a negative prognostic variable although more important as a poor prognostic factor is an antecedent hematological disturbance, that is a documented myeloid dysfunction antecedant to the transformation to acute leukemia. This factor almost certainly relates to the lack of adequate normal myeloid function which is a consequence of the dysmyelopoietic disturbance that preceded the onset of the acute leukemia transformation.

It is thus possible by a detailed analysis of variables present prior to the outset of treatment to estimate the exact probability of response for each patient with the diagnosis of adult acute leukemia and this is a technique which for us has become increasingly important in selecting primary treatment for patients with advanced metastatic disease.

Of the two-thirds or more of patients who achieve a complete remission, only one-fourth to one-fifth will enjoy prolonged survival, which is without evidence of disease for greater than three years. Thus, in our present state of knowledge, the patient in complete remission is at very high risk of recurrence, that is over 75%. Therefore this is a clinical situation which requires innovative approaches for the treatment of a patient in remission. One of the most important contributions in this field was the bone marrow transplantation studies which have indicated that with adequate intensification of therapy in first remission, patients with acute myeloblastic leukemia will rarely have recurrence of their disease. Similarly, either chemotherapy intensification early in remission or intensive intermittent reinduction over the first year of remission have both shown a disease-free survival rate which is comparable to our allogeneic bone marrow transplantation experiences at least for the first year (5). Thus it is clear that even though the patient achieves complete remission, again there is enormous heterogeneity in the likelihood that such patients can be rendered disease-free. An analysis of those variables which predict the quality of response, reveal that variables relating to the leukemia now become dominant (6). One of the most significant variables is the cytogenetic pattern of the primary acute leukemia. It has recently been possible to recognize that certain cytogenetic categories such as the 8-21 chromosome translocation or the 16 chromosome inversion abnormality are diseases where the probability of remaining in remission is excellent when compared to patients who have diploid chromosomes. In contrast to the above, cytogenetic patterns of other aneuploidies or of chromosome deletions have a particularly unfavorable likelihood of being cured after having achieved complete remission. Thus a dominant characteristic which affects the probability of cure of those patients in remission relates to the nature of the malignancy and this could never have been appreciated in the absence of treatment.

The other dominant variable in determining the quality of response is extent of disease at the time of presentation. In general, the more extensive the disease, the lower the probability of cure. In our initial studies, measurements of either lactic acid dehydrogenase in the serum or fibrinogen levels proved to be important in this regard. Recently, the lactic acid dehydrogenase data has also been reported to be prognostically significant in the cures for lymphoma. In general, for all tumors where treatment given to patients in remission is proven effective in prolonging disease-free survival, the extent of disease prior to the onset of primary treatment is the most significant variable in predicting the quality of response. Examples include the degree of lymph node involvement in breast cancer and the extent of bowel and lymph node involvement in colon cancer.

Although the underlying nature of the malignancy and the extent of disease prior to treatment dominate the ability to convert complete remission to cure, there is still an important contribution to be made by the host. In the transplant literature for instance, this is particularly striking since the likelihood of cure is inversely related to the age of the patient. In fact, most transplant centers will not undertake allogeneic bone marrow transplantation in patients over the age of 50 and since for adult acute myeloblastic leukemia, the median age in most large series is approximately 50, it means that half of the population will not tolerate the supralethal treatment required for conditioning and cytoreduction. It is almost certainly true that this is also a factor in chemotherapy intensification regimens particularly those with relatively low therapeutic indices.

2. CURRENT RESEARCH LEADS IN ACUTE LEUKEMIA

As already indicated, the study of the morphological nature of the human chromosomes has revealed changes which are of fundamental prognostic importance in human acute leukemia. Current studies of oncogenes will certainly allow a more precise definition not only of the genetic basis for this heterogeneity, but also hopefully elucidate the mechanisms for this heterogeneity by identifying gene products. The technology of cytochemistry, monoclonal antibodies, and flow microspectrophotometry (7) will surely allow a better understanding of the basis for the heterogeneity in the diseases that are lumped together as acute leukemia.

Because of the accessibility of the tumor cells in acute leukemia to the laboratory scientist, it is becoming increasingly possible to recover from both blood and bone marrow cells which can be cultivated _in vitro_. The patterns for the growth of leukemic cells _in vitro_ and particularly important, the regulation of that proliferation and differentiation _in vitro_ will almost certainly lead to a whole host of new hypotheses which can be tested _in vivo_. The field of the biological response modifiers, the lymphokines, and the macrophage originating factors will certainly provide new biologicals for clinical study. In addition, human leukemia cells have been shown to differentiate _in vitro_ in the presence of a wide array of chemical structures and biologicals. This has given rise to the hope that there will be a potential for inducing differentiation in the leukemic cells without the necessity of eradicating an entire clone of malignant cells. Some of the reports of use of low dose Ara-C provide titilating leads in that direction.

Certainly the discovery of new chemotherapeutic agents will continue to play a major role in the potential for the control of this disease and the increasing understanding of the pharmacology and biochemical mechanism of action of currently effective drugs will also almost certainly improve our therapeutic results. The reports of improved response frequencies with high dose Ara-C is a prototype for this important area of clinical study.

REFERENCES

1. Freireich EJ: Acute leukemia: A prototype of disseminated cancer. Charles F. Kettering Prize. Cancer 53:2026-2033, 1984.
2. Keating MJ, McCredie KB, Bodey GP, Smith TL, Gehan E, Freireich EJ: Improved prospects for long-term survival in adults with acute myelogenous leukemia. JAMA 248:2481-2486, 1982.
3. Keating MJ, Smith TL, Gehan EA, McCredie KB, Bodey GP, Freireich EJ: A prognostic factor analysis for use in development of predictive models for response in adult acute leukemia. Cancer 50:457-465, 1982.
4. Estey EH, Keating MJ, McCredie KB, Bodey GP, Freireich EJ: Causes of initial remission induction failure in acute myelogenous leukemia. Blood 60:309-315, 1982.
5. Zander AR, Keating M, Kanojia M, Vellekoop L, Spitzer G, Verma D, Minnhaar G, Borgelt B, Culbert S, Jagannath S, McCredie K, Freireich E, Dicke KA: Allogeneic bone marrow transplantation in acute leukemia: Piperazinedione and fractionated total body irradiation as an alternative conditioning regimen. Transplantation Proceedings 15:1392-1394, 1983.
6. Freireich EJ: Methods for evaluating response to treatment in adult acute leukemia. Blood Cells 9:5-20, 1983.
7. Barlogie B, Raber MN, Schumann J, Johnson TS, Drewinko B, Swartzendruber DE, Gohde W, Andreeff M, Freireich EJ: Flow cytometry in clinical cancer research. Cancer Res. 43:3982-3997, 1983.

2

EXPERIMENTAL RATIONALE FOR THERAPY IN THE TREATMENT OF ACUTE LEUKEMIA

Frederick A. Valeriote, Ph.D.

1. INTRODUCTION

The treatment of human leukemia from a scientific approach marks its beginnings from the mid 1950's with the establishment of a group of clinicians at the National Cancer Institute which included Drs. Frei, Holland, Zubrod and Freireich. Concomitant with the establishment of this clinical program was the development of at least 3 major experimental programs: two in experimental therapeutics headed by Dr. Abraham Goldin at the NCI and Dr. Howard Skipper at Southern Research Institute, and one in pharmacology under Dr. Rall at the NCI. The history of these groups and cross-fertilization of concepts between the laboratory and the clinic has become a model for the interaction between bench and clinical investigators (1). I will attempt here to review some facets of the role played by experimentalists such as these using leukemia models in the development of a scientific approach to human leukemia therapy.

A major problem with trying to pinpoint the importance and application of experimental leukemia models to the understanding and treatment of human leukemia, however, results from the pervasiveness of experimental leukemias in cancer research. This is unlike nearly every other tumor system where specific similarities between the experimental model and the clinical tumor are the basis for their study. However, the ease of study and relative simplicity of leukemia lines have attracted investigators to use leukemia models to answer questions on cancer in general and not leukemia in particular. Indeed, it is fortunate that much of the information obtained has had applicability not only to our understanding of the disease process of cancer in general, but also to the treatment for human leukemia in particular.

Nearly every aspect of cancer biology has made use of leukemia models. Radiation leukemogenesis was an early experimental finding in mice which provided an understanding of radiation as an underlying causative factor in leukemia. Animal studies led to the discovery of the murine leukemia viruses which have had a major impact in Biology with the discovery of RNA dependent DNA polymerase (2), the importance of viruses as causative agents in cancer (3), the development of the oncogene theory and the rationale for the present findings on human leukemia viruses (4) as discussed by Dr. Golde in this Symposium. The finding of tumor specific antigens, initially as expressions of tumorigenic viruses, of normal cell markers such as theta antigen and surface immunoglobulin led to a dramatic expansion of research on tumor markers with the present antigenic markers in leukemias serving an increasingly important diagnostic and potential therapeutic role as discussed by both Palutke and Foon in this Symposium.

In cancer chemotherapy, most studies on the mechanism of action of agents have been done on leukemia models. Two examples of many are the landmark studies from Hall's laboratory defining sensitivity of cells in terms of specific activating enzymes (5), and the recent work of Kohn and others with alkaline elution techniques to determine the various interactions of alkylating agents with DNA (6). This sensitive technique of alkaline elution may provide us with a way of determining prior to treatment the sensitivity of a given patient's tumor to a variety of DNA binders and alkylating agents. Indeed, most of the presentations in this Symposium probably take as their starting point, or rely heavily upon, basic studies utilizing leukemia models.

As Zubrod recently pointed out (7), in the initial development of the NCI program, L1210 leukemia was chosen as the model for childhood ALL. The present 50% cure rate for ALL in children and 15% cure rate in adults owes much to the clinical application of concepts derived from experimental studies on this and other leukemia models. I have chosen to discuss here a number of the concepts which I believe are important to Oncology in general, therapy in particular and which have developed from studies with experimental leukemias. As I discuss each of the topics, I will also indicate how future studies might be expected to contribute to both our knowledge and therapy.

2. DRUG SCREENING AND MECHANISM OF ACTION

From the beginning of the drug screening program to the present time at both the National Cancer Institute and at drug companies, experimental leukemias have been the main, if not the sole, prescreen. This prescreen selects those agents which are to be used not only for the treatment of leukemia but, more importantly, in the treatment of all human cancers (8). It is therefore legitimate to emphasize that the success of the present therapy of leukemia rests on the past discoveries of agents from these leukemia screens. Indeed, the rationale in the selection of anticancer agents is that they must be cytotoxic to experimental leukemia cells. If they are not so cytotoxic, they are excluded from further study. It is fair to state that such agents are invariably anti-proliferative rather than specifically anti-leukemic and obviously the former is the reason for any activity against solid tumors.

As to future studies, while it seems reasonable to include solid tumors into the prescreen when possible, there remains a need for effective anticancer agents for the treatment of leukemia. Therefore the leukemia prescreens can be expected to continue to provide new agents to the clinic.

A second major use of these leukemia models has been to examine the mechanism of action of the clinically active anticancer agents. From transport of alkylating agents (9), to activation of nucleosides (10), interaction of active species with target enzyme (11), or interaction of agents with DNA (12), leukemia cells have been and remain the cell type from which such basic information is obtained. Indeed, we have only begun to understand the biochemical mechanism of action of most agents, especially as to how the biochemical effect relates to cytotoxicity. As a single example, the most potent class of lympholytic agents are the corticosteroids, specifically prednisone and prednisolone. They are probably the least understood of the anticancer agents used. Further studies on their mechanism of action is required including the role of receptors in the target cells (13,14), the mechanism of resistance development (15) and their modulating effect on normal and tumor cell proliferation (16).

We can expect increasing amounts of important information on drug action to continue to be derived from leukemia models.

3. TREATMENT WITH SINGLE AGENTS

3.1 Scheduling studies

In the early 1950's Goldin's group employed the L1210 leukemia as a model for human leukemia to begin studies on the antitumor effect of single agents, initially aminopterin and amethopterin. They developed the still-standard practice of examining the effect of a range of i.p. doses of the given drug a few days following the i.p. inoculation of tumor cells on increase in lifespan of the treated mice (compared to untreated controls). Further, they began the practice of examining a variety of treatment schedules within a given study. Their initial studies with methotrexate (Figure 1A) led to the proposal that this agent should be administered in an intermittent schedule (17).

Further studies of Goldin with methotrexate led to the important finding that the stage of the disease can influence significantly the optimal schedule. For later stage L1210 leukemia, daily administration of drug was most effective (Figure 1B) (18). Such results have been taken into consideration when dealing with induction therapy where there is a large tumor mass compared to maintenance therapy in which case many fewer cells exist in the host (19). Present-day chemotherapy, however, involves multiple agents simultaneously and their interactions become increasingly important (20).

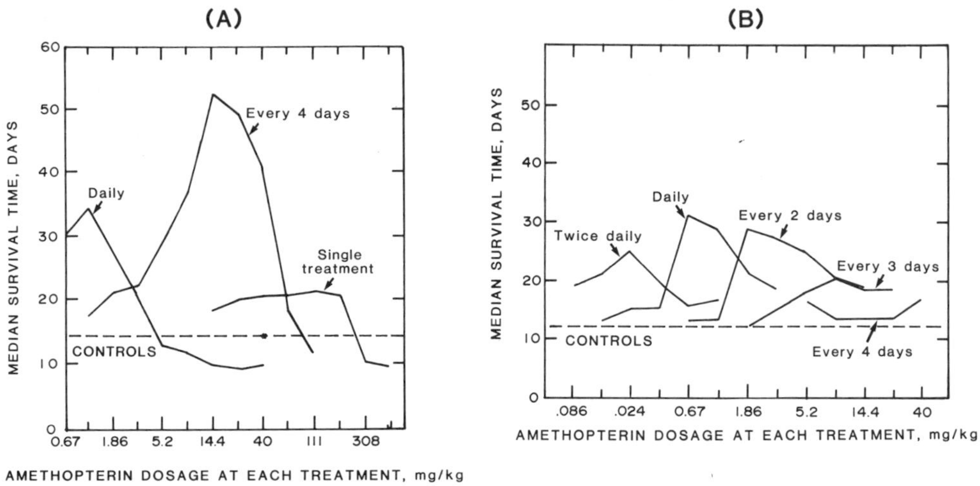

Figure 1. Median survival time of mice bearing L1210 leukemia with Amethopterin treatment begun A) 5 days or B) 8 days after leukemia cell inoculation. Results taken from Ref. 17 and 18, respectively.

These type of scheduling studies, however, are invariably carried out in experimental leukemia models for all anticancer agents before they reach clinical trial (21), the results of which are a factor in determining the appropriate clinical schedule for a given agent.

3.2 Dose-survival relationships

Goldin et al (22) were first to demonstrate the important dose-response relationship in which higher doses of amethopterin were required to cure mice of increasing leukemia cell burdens. However, this concept received its greatest impact with the development of quantitative assays first for tissue cultured mammalian cells and later for leukemia cells _in vivo_ (23,24). While the initial studies were based upon radiation effects, the importance of the relationship for alkylating agents and other anticancer agents both to understand and plan therapy soon became evident (25,26). Till and McCullock used the same concept to obtain the first dose-response curve for normal tissue _in vivo_ (27).

With the development of quantitative assessment of tumor cell survival either by mouse survival time or clonogenic assays, the exponential $[S=(N/No)e^{-\alpha D}]$ relationship for a number of anticancer agents was discovered. For agents other than the phase-specific ones, for example, with the alkylating agents, quantitative studies demonstrated a direct relationship of dose and cell survival, and Skipper termed this first-order killing (28). In Figure 2, I have presented this relationship for a variety of anticancer agents on two standard leukemia models. The observation by myself and others that increasing drug dose leads to increasing cell destruction has become the basis for the use of large, intermittent doses of anticancer agents. Further, because of the steepness of the dose-survival curves for many agents, a small increase in dose can be translated to a large increase in cell killing.

Indeed, this relationship is the basis for the Phase I clinical studies of defining the maximum tolerated dose for subsequent clinical protocols.

Frei recently pointed out (29) that a dose-response relationship has become gospel in Radiotherapy leading to the presently used high, often locally curative, doses. Indeed, Kaplan noted nearly two decades ago the relationship between dose and local recurrence rate following irradiation (30). For clinical chemotherapy studies, however, there are relatively few studies which have been carried out to demonstrate this relationship, but when done it is usually noted that any significant reduction in dose will compromise response rates (29).

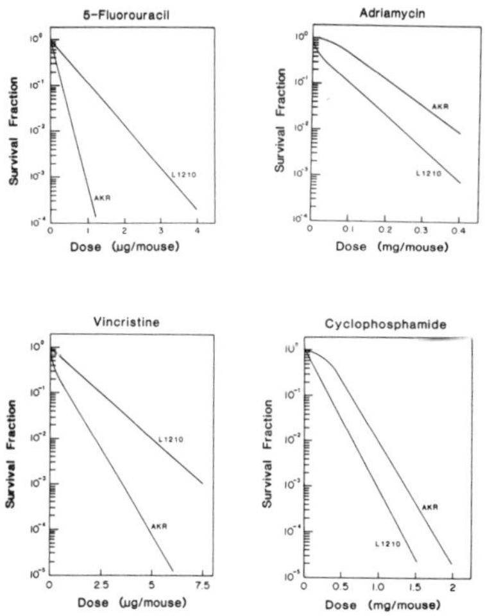

Figure 2. Dose-survival relationship of AKR and L1210 leukemia cells to different anticancer agents.

Pinkel et al (31) examined this question of the dose-response relationship for childhood lymphocytic leukemia using a 4-drug antileukemic combination at either full or half dose. They showed a striking difference for duration of both complete remission and hematologic remission as well as for survival with the full dose group being significantly better. However, it should be noted that relapse was mainly CNS disease which occurred much earlier in the half versus full dose group (4 months versus 10 months).

An obvious corollary of this concept was deduced by Skipper (28) (Figure 3) of remission duration being proportional to tumor cell killing. This obviously has application in the clinical philosophy that one progresses from increasing the proportions of complete remissions to increasing the duration of remissions and finally to cures. In fact, clinicians have used this concept to estimate the residual leukemia cell burden in patients following therapy based on their remission duration (32).

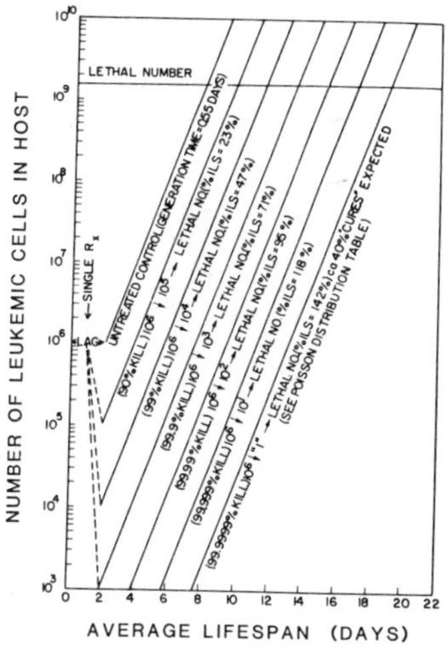

Figure 3. Correlation of survival time with percentage of leukemia cell kill. Taken from Ref. 28.

One group of agents did not follow an exponential dose-response relationship but yielded plateau-type dose-response curves. They have been termed phase-specific agents because they exerted their cytotoxic effect in some specific (usually S) phase of the cell cycle. Since the optimal use of such agents would be to expose the cells to cytotoxic concentrations over a period of time so as to allow all of the tumor cells to traverse the sensitive phase of the cell cycle in the presence of lethal drug concentration, these results have led to the scheduling of agents such as cytosine arabinoside either as an infusion or by repeated, short interval administrations (33,34). Figure 4 demonstrates this effect where single dose and infused dose of ara-C are compared. Subsequent clinical studies demonstrated the efficacy of infusional ara-C in cancer (35).

While the greater effectiveness of the infusion schedule seems plain, it is necessary to realize that host toxicity is also increased with the infusion schedule. Indeed, for ara-C the experimental leukemia model shows little if any difference in therapeutic effectiveness for infusional ara-C versus high dose, bolus ara-C.

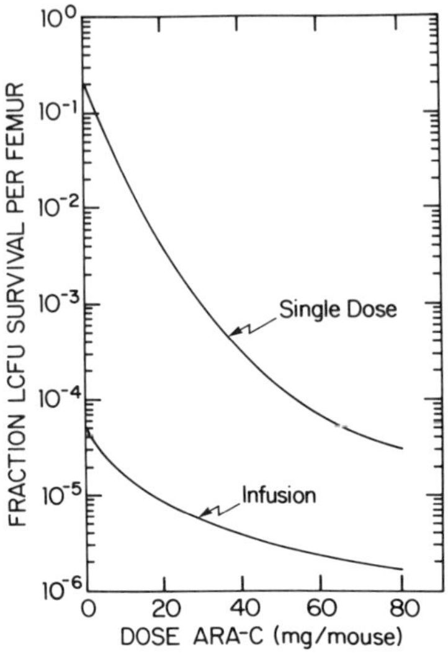

Figure 4. Survival of leukemia cells as a function of ara-C dose for either bolus or infused schedule. Taken from Ref. 34.

Scheduling studies will continue in the future with all new investigational drugs in murine leukemia models as well as in Phase I studies to provide direction in Phase II and III clinical studies. I believe that more in-depth experimental and clinical studies on bolus versus infusion scheduling are also necessary.

3.3 Clonogenicity of leukemia

The concept of clonogenicity has had a major impact upon our ideas about leukemia therapy. The fact that a single, clonogenic cell if left in the host can proliferate and kill the host is an important concept proposed first by Furth (36) and expanded upon in Skipper's studies (28). It played a major role in the development of intensive clinical antileukemia therapy with complete eradication of the disease; that is, the killing of every leukemia cell as the goal of therapy. This has guided present-day clinical therapy with regard to treatment of patients in remission since leukemia can regrow from a single surviving cell and thus all tumor cells must be destroyed if cure is to be obtained. Indeed, the continued treatment of patients even after complete remission is obtained results from the understanding that the two or three decades of tumor cell killing necessary to produce a complete remission is but the first stage (the induction phase) in the goal of tumor eradication.

However, the concept of having to kill the last malignant cell may also be an artifact of studies with experimental leukemias. These tumors generally have little if any immunologic component and also a high proportion of the cells are malignant or clonogenic - i.e. have extensive proliferative capacity. This may not represent the biological situation in human leukemias where only a small fraction of the tumor cells are clonogenic.

One area of study which approaches this question of the size of the clonogenic cell population is that of the human tumor stem cell assay. While this technique has been popularized for the examination of drug sensitivity profiles for tumors of individual patients (37), its use is having a major impact upon our understanding of the biology of both normal and malignant neoplasms (38). It is interesting to note that while experimental leukemias such as L1210 were readily cloned *in vitro* many years ago, and that a major impetus to this field resulted from the laboratory plasmacytoma studies (39,40) which led to the initial work on human myeloma (41), unfortunately, clonogenic studies on human leukemias have been outpaced by the success with cloning of solid tumors. However, advances are being made in this area such as the studies of Buick (42) which indicate that important questions on the biology of the leukemia cell can be answered. The work of Priesler (43) shows the potential of this assay for predictive chemotherapy response. Future manipulations *in vitro* of the chemical environment of a given patient's tumor cells may also be employed to indicate optimal therapy.

4. RADIATION THERAPY

Radiation therapy is a major branch of Oncology with a strong experimental base having an important, though limited role in the treatment of leukemias. A number of our concepts in tumor therapy has resulted from basic studies in this field. The first *in vivo* quantitation of the lethal effect of radiation on mammalian cells was carried out by Hewitt on a leukemia cell line (24). The dose-survival curve was interesting in relation to both parameters which describe radiation dose-survival curves. The slope of the dose-response curve yielded a D_0 value of about 115 rads and an "n" value was about 1.6. In subsequent radiation studies with hematological tumors, even smaller D_0 values have been reported and n values of 1 or less noted (44,45,46). Figure 5 presents some information from the literature which indicates this situation. The low D_0 value indicates the intrinsic sensitivity of the tumor to radiation while the low n value implies that the killing efficiency of even the smallest dose of radiation is similar to that noted at higher doses. This relatively radiation-sensitive state for hematological tumors appears to hold also for the cell of origin - the hematopoietic stem cell (27).

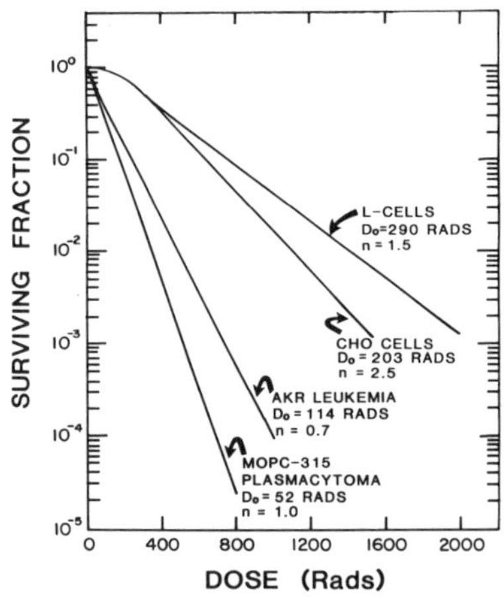

Figure 5. Radiation dose-survival curves for different mammalian cells.

Normal cells or cells from non-hematological tumors, however, though highly variable, have D_O values in the order of 150 rads and extrapolation numbers greater than 1.5 (47-51).

One might then extrapolate these results to the clinic and implicate radiation as an obvious and important modality for the treatment of leukemias. Indeed, irradiation of hematological tumors either as solid masses as in plasmacytomas or areas of accumulation of tumor cells as in lymphomas and CLL, or in locations where chemotherapy entry is limited such as the CNS, has become standard practice. However, the disseminated nature of leukemia limits the use of radiation therapy.

While there is little ongoing research in radiotherapy or radiobiology directly related to leukemia, some of the present exciting research in this area, such as with sensitizers, protectors and hyperthermia, may have important applications in the therapy of leukemia. For example, we have demonstrated that the radiation protector WR-2721 can protect normal tissue from the cytotoxic effect of nitrogen mustard while it concomitantly potentiates the cytotoxicity of leukemia cells to nitrogen mustard (52). Whether this finding will have applicability in human leukemia awaits further study.

A similar situation exists for radiation sensitizers in that sensitization of the cytotoxicity of alkylating agents seems to occur for leukemia cells (53). In fact, it is likely that interactions noted with radiation for sensitizers, potentiators or thiol manipulators in general can be translatable to similar interactions with alkylating agents with possible application to leukemia therapy.

Finally, the new modality of hyperthermia which is an important new potential for radiation therapy may have similarly important implications for medical oncology. Sapareto (54) (Figure 6) has shown that leukemias are more sensitive than normal stem cells to hyperthermia and possibly T-cell leukemias in general are very sensitive. Thus hyperthermia may have clinical applicability to the leukemia patient either directly by whole-body heating or indirectly by purging isologous marrow transplants of leukemia cells.

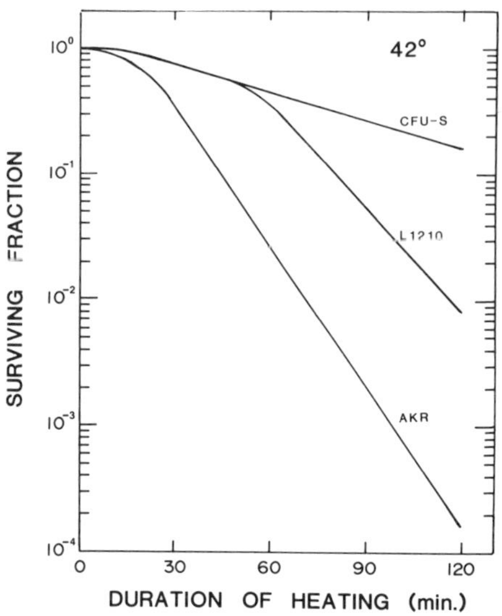

Figure 6. Survival of 3 different cell populations as a function of heating duration at 42° *in vitro*. Results taken from Ref. 54.

5. COMBINATION CHEMOTHERAPY

Research on possible additive or synergistic effects of anticancer agents using experimental leukemias was begun in the late 1940's (55); and, with the increase in the number of active agents, has become a major area of research investigation. Obviously from nitrogen mustard in 1946 and Amethopterin in 1948 to the present 3 dozen or so clinically useful agents plus the investigational agents, a strong scientific rationale is a requisite in obtaining optimal two-, three- or multi-drug combinations.

It seemed obvious early in both experimental and clinical studies (32) that combinations of agents were more effective than single agents. While studies on drug combinations in both experimental and clinical settings often appeared more empirical than scientific, a number of basic concepts have been developed and applied as the scientific rationale for combination therapy. These were:

a) OVERCOME RESISTANCE DEVELOPMENT.
b) NON-OVERLAPPING HOST TOXICITIES.
c) SYNCHRONIZATION OF TUMOR CELLS.
d) RECRUITMENT OF TUMOR CELLS.
e) OBTAIN BIOCHEMICAL SYNERGISM.
f) BIOCHEMICAL MODULATION.

Each of these concepts are discussed below.

Two-drug combinations were first examined in the early days of experimental chemotherapy with the idea of controlling the development of drug resistance following single agent therapy (56), however, it became obvious that positive (synergistic) interactions could occur between agents to increase their effectiveness (57). This led to extensive studies over the years examining nearly every conceivable two-drug combination for interaction as generally defined in terms of increased survival time of leukemia-bearing mice.

Goldin's group introduced the practice of studying the effect of drug combinations on host toxicity concomitant with the tumor studies (58). In this way they could determine whether therapeutic synergism occurred with a given combination. Indeed, the importance of this was demonstrated by the fine studies of Schabel's group indicating that for many combinations one observes less than additive toxicity of the agents (59). My laboratory has expanded on these studies by examining the parameters of sequence and interval dependency for two drug combinations. There are many combinations which we have found to yield synergistic cytotoxic interactions when the two agents are separated by an interval of time such as Ara-C and Daunorubicin (60) or Vincristine and Cyclophosphamide (61). And alternatively, there are combinations which demonstrate a synergistic interaction when administered close in time such as Cyclophosphamide and BCNU (62) or Ara-C and MTX (63).

From the beginning of combination chemotherapy research studies, there has been two major directions - one attempting to employ principles of cell kinetics and the second attempting a biochemical approach to both define and explain the experimental findings.

5.1 Cell kinetic factors

Two areas of cell kinetic application in leukemia relate to synchronization and recruitment. Much of the early studies on synchronization were done *in vitro*, in normal tissues and in both murine leukemias and solid tumors (64) and demonstrated the potential of this approach.

An example of a rational application of concepts of tumor cell synchronization in experimental studies to therapy can be shown for S-phase specific agents which kill only proliferating cells during one portion of the cell cycle. It obviously would not be reasonable to administer two such agents, at full doses, at the same time. Indeed experimental studies in mice showed that for ara-C and thiopurines, a period of time in the order of 10 to 20 hours was necessary (Figure 7). Obviously, for such a strategy to be effective one needs to have knowledge on parameters such as whether the cells are sensitive to both agents and the rate of refilling of the sensitive phase.

This approach to drug scheduling has been used in the treatment of leukemia with Ara-C and thioguanine. Indeed, in our study we noted that simultaneous Ara-C and TG was less effective than TG alone. This was likely due to inhibition of DNA synthesis by Ara-C resulting in TG not being incorporated into DNA. The specific clinical studies did not follow from this but preceeded the animal studies using the identical rationale of overlapping phase sensitivities (65) and was found useful in ALL (66).

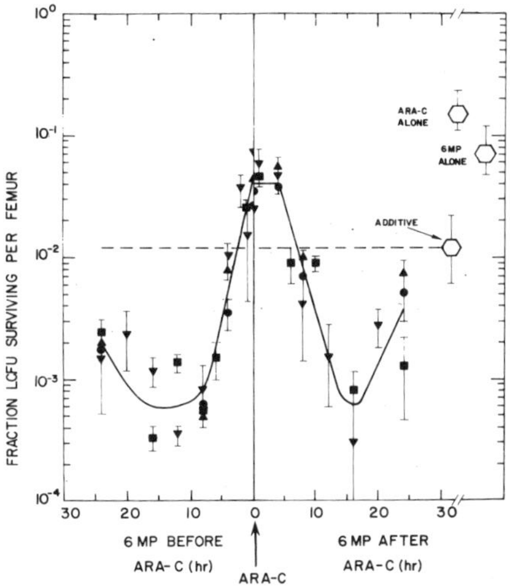

Figure 7. Survival of leukemia cells for different sequences and intervals for Ara-C and 6MP.

There have been a few clinical studies, many with leukemias, which have attempted to develop this potential application of synchronization. Most studies have seemed inconclusive although some positive results have been noted, such as the studies of Klein (67).

The second area, that of cell recruitment, has been actively pursued in experimental models as well as clinical studies. Schabel first proposed this in experimental studies with a plasmacytoma where the first course of therapy recruited non-proliferating cells into cell cycle and the subsequent therapy was active against the cycling cells (68).

In human leukemia it is known that a fraction of the malignant cells can be non-proliferating but capable of re-entering cell cycle (69). In dealing with the question of recruitment, however, the standard transplantable tumors are not useful since few if any of their clonogenic cells are in a non-proliferating state except in the far-advanced disease state. A reasonable candidate for such studies is the spontaneous lymphoma model in AKR mice. Indeed, a finding noted early by Rosen et al (70) using spontaneous AKR lymphoma was the existence of small, non-proliferating blast cells with potential proliferative capacity (tumor G_0 cells).

Investigators, such as Burke, have attempted to use drug scheduling to force such non-proliferating cells into cycle followed by cytotoxic therapy at an optimal time thereafter to maximize tumor cell killing. They have employed a rat leukemia model as the basis for subsequent clinical trials (71,72).

A major technical limitation in the studies on both synchronization and recruitment has been the lack of a rapid and sensitive means of defining the cell cycle location of clonogenic cells at any given time. However, one can now employ flow cytometry to define the effectiveness of synchronization and recruitment strategies (possibly in combination with clonogenic assays) so as to define optimal drug timing. It seems imperative that future studies on synchronization be specifically directed to the clonogenic cells since these cells are the obvious target of the therapy. Indeed, until we can obtain accurate information on clonogenic cell fraction, cell cycle times and their distributions, growth fraction and recruitment rates from non-proliferating compartments following therapy, our ability to employ the experimentally-derived concepts of synchronization and recruitment will remain coarse.

The purpose of discussing these combinations is that strategies can be developed and tested experimentally. Cellular and biochemical rationales can be readily tested and while the list of such possible studies is enormous, one example would be to examine experimentally the TAD (6-thioguanine, Ara-C, Daunorubicin) combination used in AML. Dose, schedule, sequence and interval could be readily modified and studied. Those rationales which work in animal models would then be appropriate Phase II selections.

5.2 Biochemical modulation

An increasingly important subject deals with the manipulation of the biochemical reactions within the normal or tumor cell with usually non-toxic agents so as to make the cell either more or less sensitive to exposure to a subsequent cytotoxic anticancer agent. Probably the early studies of Goldin in which leucovorin was used to limit the cytotoxicity of amethopterin on L1210 leukemia cells was the first such attempt (73). This work led to the use of high dose methotrexate in clinical studies with leucovorin rescue.

We pursued the use of thymidine and other normal DNA and RNA substrates to modify the cytotoxic activity of 5-fluorouracil (FUra) against AKR leukemia cells and observed that optimal scheduling of these agents produced a large increase in tumor cell killing (74,75). The potentiation noted has led to the study of a host of biochemical modulators in leukemia and other tumors with FUra and other antimetabolites such as Ara-C.

Future studies can be expected to be more extensive and more sophisticated, for example, manipulating the thiol content of cells to make them more or less sensitive to anticancer agents.

Finally, while the above area of research has dealt with the use of non-cytotoxic agents in combination with cytotoxic agents, there have also been many studies where one anticancer agent itself is employed to modulate the cellular response to a second cytotoxic agent. An example of this direction is with combination FUra and MTX as studied by Cadman (76) whereby MTX pretreatment is able to increase the formation of FUra ribonucleotides and subsequent cellular cytotoxicity.

6. IMPORTANCE OF THE BLOOD-BRAIN BARRIER

The importance of CNS leukemia in both the natural history of the disease and as a major limitation in effective chemotherapy was recognized early in the treatment of leukemia (77,78). The major clinical advance resulted when the combination of radiation and intrathecal MTX demonstrated good control of this problem with significant extension of continuous complete remission (79).

Skipper and others demonstrated a number of years ago that agents such as cyclophosphamide could destroy all leukemia cells systemically but had little effect on the cells which had migrated to and were growing in the central nervous system (80). The killing of intracerebrally-innoculated leukemia cells was used as a model in a synthesis program to develop agents which crossed the blood-brain barrier; a striking outcome was the alkylating nitrosoureas which were synthesized specifically to cross the blood-brain barrier and destroy leukemia cells (81). This model was also employed to demonstrate the utility of radiation plus cytotoxic agents (82) against CNS leukemia.

This problem of CNS disease continues (83) and probably will be resolved with the introduction of new agents possibly selected by an experimental CNS leukemia model. Our limited work in this area has demonstrated that this disease can be attacked and successfully eradicated in a murine model by a systemically developed anti-tumor immune response (84).

7. NORMAL HEMATOPOIESIS AND LEUKEMIA

For many investigators involved in research with leukemia models, some component of their research has often involved the hematopoietic system. Thus it would seem incomplete if some comment were not made upon the research on this, the normal counterpart of the leukemia model. Ideas on cell kinetics, cell control, differentiation, oncogenesis and therapy have developed from the intensive concurrent research carried out on the normal hematopoietic system. Many of these studies have had an impact on leukemia biology.

7.1 The hematopoietic stem cell

A major concept in leukemia biology which is basic to therapy philosophy is that of the normal stem cell. The functional demonstration and quantitation by Till and McCulloch (85) in normal hematopoietic tissue has made it and its clonogenic descendents a major locus for research activity related to therapy. Numerous studies of drug and radiation sensitivity have been carried out on the two physiological states of this cell - the G_0 and proliferative state. Two scientific tenets for therapy scheduling are that drugs are more toxic to proliferating cells (86), and that a depletion of the descendent hematopoietic cells leads to the recruitment of non-proliferating stem cells into cycle and their subsequent sensitization. As demonstrated in experimental animals (87) with subsequent repopulation of the hematopoietic tissues following therapy the stem cells revert to a less sensitive, non-proliferative state. The limitation in continuous treatment and the requirement for 3 to 4 weeks of rest between high dose therapy has the above as its scientific basis.

Further, a major advance in Cell Biology resulted from the *in vitro* cloning of normal committed hematopoietic stem cells by Bradley and Metcalf (88). This technique has been employed by numerous investigators to examine the biology of the normal hematopoietic system and presaged the development of colony assays for leukemia cells of both experimental animals and humans.

7.2 Differentiation of normal and leukemic cells

Certainly much of the information learned about regulation of the hematopoietic system has had an impact on the ideas of differentiation abnormalities as an underlying cellular cause of leukemia. The complexity of the regulatory system for proliferation and differentiation has led to the proposal as shown in Figure 8 that the malignant transformation occurs early in the myeloid differentiation sequence, in erythroblasts for erythroleukemia and the lymphoblast for ALL. Further, defects in either or both proliferative and differentiation controls have been proposed and the elegant work of Sachs (89) with experimental leukemia has provided important basic knowledge concerning tumor cell regulation as well as a potential approach to therapy. For example, Sachs has shown that myeloid leukemia cells respond to presumably normal growth regulators such as MGI (macrophage and granulocyte inducer) (90).

The possibility of using factors to allow or force terminal differentiation of the malignant cell is highlighted in the work of investigators such as Bloch (91), as described by him in this Symposium, who attempt to restore order to this disorder in myelopoiesis not only through phenotype modulation but also by repressing oncogene transcription (Figure 8). A most interesting recent observation from such studies is that cytotoxic agents such as cytosine arabinoside can produce such terminal differentiation. Indeed, striking therapeutic responses have already been noted in the treatment of leukemias using low dose schedules attempting to induce terminal differentiation (92).

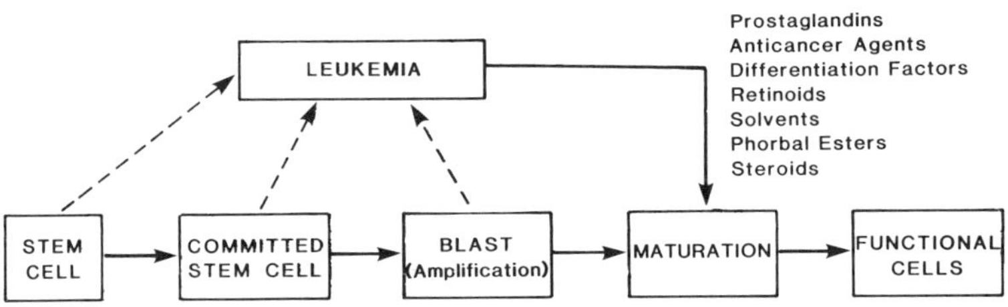

Figure 8. Schematic representation of malignant transformation in the myeloid pathway and factors which can lead to differentiation of the leukemia cells.

The inhibitory effect of leukemia cells on normal bone marrow is probably of great significance for intensive induction therapy. The expanding leukemia clone appears to produce normal inhibitory substances (lactoferrin) (93) and may even inhibit normal myelopoiesis by cell contact. This has a positive effect for successful therapy since we know from experimental models that if the residual stem cells were all in cycle as a response to the depleted functional cellular elements which occurs with advancing leukemia, then their drug sensitivity would be markedly increased and the extent of therapy dramatically curtailed. Since this likely is not the situation and the stem cells are in a drug-protected physiological state then the standard intensive, rapid therapy of agents with limited cytotoxicity to stem cells is appropriate and obviously effective in induction therapy (94).

A major advance in experimental hematology has been the development of a long term _in vitro_ system which mimics the _in vivo_ situation - the so-called Dexter system (95). This culture not only allows us to study normal hematopoiesis but also the transformed state as Hines points out in this Symposium.

7.3 Bone marrow transplantation

Even though many agents demonstrate some degree of selectivity to tumor cells, for radiation and a number of chemotherapeutic agents there often is no selectivity (26,96). However, this "problem" can be made use of in the therapy of leukemia in the case of bone marrow transplantation.

Lorenz et al (97) demonstrated over 30 years ago that marrow injected into lethally irradiated mice could protect them from death. This observation has become the basis for marrow transplantation following intensive chemotherapy (98). While animal studies will continue to define procedures to optimally ablate the recipient's immune system, the problem of graft-versus-host disease (GVHD) requires investigation not only in terms of the cellular basis of its response but also on means for its abrogation. One area of future potential is hyperthermia. If this heat response sensitivity shown by T-cell tumors indicated previously (Figure 6) is demonstrated by normal T-cells as well, then it may be a procedure of abrogating GVHD by pre-heating marrow before transplantation.

One proposal, made nearly 20 years ago, was to emphasize "methods of protecting the patient from the toxic effect of antileukemic agents thus allowing for the delivery of larger doses" (32). While the use of supportive techniques such as transfusion therapy has had some impact, as discussed by Karanes in this Symposium, possibly some of the newer procedures of cellular sulfhydryl level manipulation will be of future use.

8. IMMUNOTHERAPY

One area of cancer research which certainly has had its ups and downs over the last decade is immunotherapy. While individuals may disagree on its exact beginnings, certainly the work of Mathe with transplantable leukemias employing BCG (99) (Figure 9) led to a burst of activity with translation to many clinical protocols (100). A concept which developed from these early studies was that immunotherapy would be successful only for minimal residual disease (<10^6 malignant cells) (101). This logically led to immunochemotherapy protocols in which the tumor cellularity was first decreased by chemotherapy and then followed by immunotherapy (102), and also to the study of a host of immune stimulators including tumor cells (irradiated or treated with neuraminidase), C. parvum, polymers, and even graft-versus-leukemia models. Indeed, it seemed that in the mid-70's every second protocol in Cooperative Group studies had an immunotherapy or chemoimmunotherapy arm.

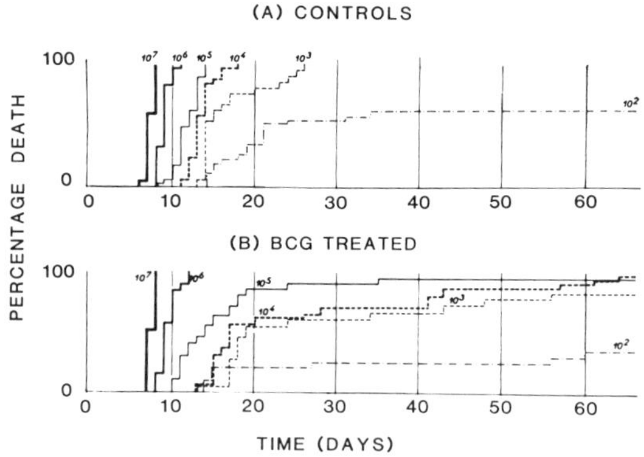

Figure 9. Survival of mice bearing different inocula of L1210 cells. A) Control and B) BCG-treated. Redrawn from Ref. 99.

However, studies such as ours indicated that an immune reaction can develop in a "syngeneic" murine model leading to the rejection of 10^{10} leukemia cells (103). The results presented in Figure 10 show the kinetics of this response in mice bearing an advanced leukemia and treated with Amphotericin B plus BCNU. Further studies showed that this immunologic response did not occur for minimal disease (104). In Figure 10 the kinetics of an allograft rejection is shown for comparison (105). Once immunity has been established it can seemingly take care of grams of cells with ease.

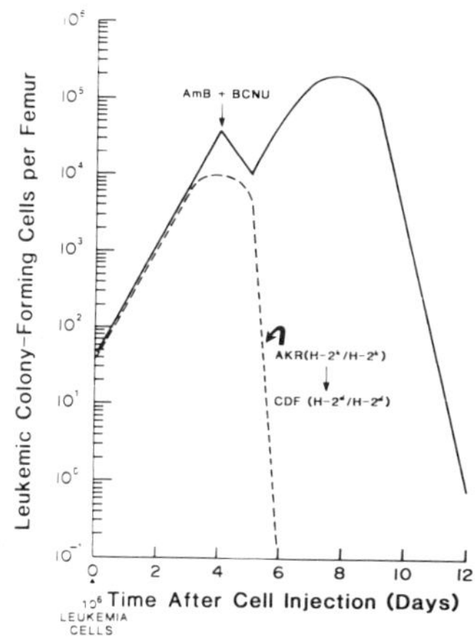

Figure 10. Kinetics of leukemia cell rejection in a model for chemoimmunotherapy (solid line, taken from Ref. 103). Also shown (dashed line) is the kinetics of leukemia cell rejection across a major histocompatibility locus (taken from Ref. 105).

Beside models in which the immune system of the host is modified to attack resident tumor cells, evidence exists that the host's immune system normally can regulate tumor cell growth and differentiation. The example of the murine plasmacytomas has been well documented in that regard (106). Such "natural" regulation of human hematological tumors is a potential area for future study on which to devise possible immunological therapeutic interventions.

Immunotherapy, both active and passive, is presently going through a resurgence and it is hoped that application of interferons or monoclonals will have therapeutic application as discussed by Foon in this Symposium. While exciting results in human lymphoma has recently demonstrated the potential of monoclonal therapy, the specificity of such therapy may itself be a limitation. The spontaneous AKR leukemia has been shown to be composed of at least four antigenically different subpopulations and requires at least four different monoclonals for complete cure of the mice (107). This heterogeneous nature of tumor cells first demonstrated with murine mammary tumors (108) appears to be re-affirmed in murine lymphomas and leukemias and of significant importance in both the biology of the disease and its therapy. Use of interleukins in developing T-cell clones for passive, adoptive immunotherapy is an experimentally promising development which has high specificity, allows use of syngeneic cells, and allows a "reagent" approach to immunotherapy by chosen, pure T-cell subsets. Present major studies in this area employ a lymphoma model (109).

9. RESISTANCE

Resistance to therapy is a major factor limiting successful cure of leukemia. Resistance can develop through a variety of mechanisms, and indeed, for a given agent, any step from crossing the cell membrane to the final moment when the cell is biologically dead, mechanisms can intervene to protect the cell (110). Leukemia cell models have been employed extensively to define resistance mechanisms and Figure 11 presents a comprehensive up-to-date schematic of the cellular processes involved. While investigators have made use of cells other than leukemia cells for studies on drug resistance, including CHO, L, HeLa and Ehrlich ascites cells as Kessel discusses in this Symposium, leukemia cells have been instrumental in unravelling this fundamental problem as well as providing clues to methods for overcoming the resistance. Leukemia models have demonstrated both decreased drug uptake (111) as well as gene amplification (11) for resistance to methotrexate. The former might be overcome by lipid soluble antifolates and the latter by high dose methotrexate. Increased efflux has been noted for Adriamycin (112) and efflux inhibitors proposed to overcome the resistance. And, finally target competitors have been implicated in melphalan resistance (113) with agents which decrease glutathione as likely candidates for modifiers of this state.

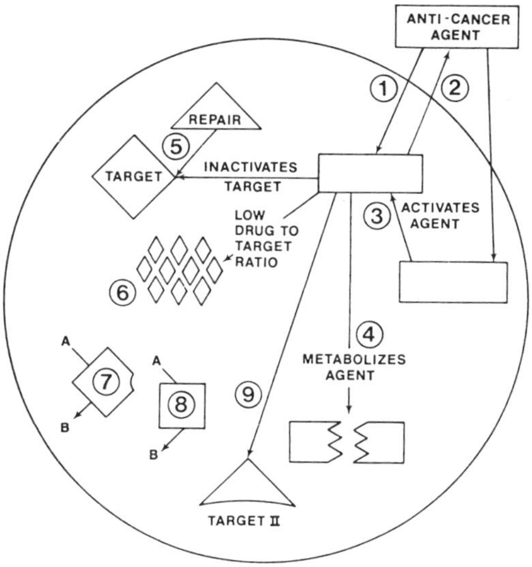

Figure 11. Different possible mechanisms by which a cell can become resistant to anticancer agents:

1) decreased uptake
2) increased efflux
3) decreased activation
4) increased inactivation
5) repair of lesion
6) increased synthesis of targets
7) decreased binding to target
8) development of alternate pathway
9) production of different targets

While future studies will continue to make use of leukemia models to determine the biochemical basis of resistance, one should expect that an increasing number of studies will be directed at circumventing such resistance. Indeed, recent examples of such an approach include the use of calcium channel blockers such as verapamil to reverse adriamycin resistance (114) or polyenes such as Amphotericin B to reverse resistance to Actinomycin D (115).

10. CONCLUSION

Hopefully, I have demonstrated the importance of murine leukemia models in the development of cancer therapy. These models have had a major impact on the concepts and therapy of cancer in general and I expect will remain a major resource for such studies in the future. These models will be employed to examine mechanisms of leukemogenesis, to search for new drugs, to analyze combination therapies, to study the control of growth and differentiation and to define both the basis of drug resistance and interventions to abrogate the resistance. However, with the development of tissue culture technology and better understanding of <u>in vitro</u> growth regulation, an increasing number of human cell lines, such as K562 (116), will be employed to study the above questions. While I have indicated ongoing or future research with these experimental models, there are many areas which I did not touch upon, for example, NMR analysis of ^{31}P or ^{13}C spectra following cell exposure to candidate anticancer agents or use of flow cytometry for fluorescent anticancer agents such as the anthracyclines to define drug sensitivity.

I have possibly over-emphasized the importance of murine leukemia models in the success story to date for treatment of human leukemias; however, their importance is indeed beyond question. Certainly much of clinical therapy is empirical and a good idea on the part of an academic clinician has been as important in advancing treatment results as any single application of an experimental study. Indeed, the flow of ideas between the two is essential since a major problem with the experimental animal models is their homogenization of the factors being studied. As an example of this, Freireich dramatically points out in this Symposium, both the existence and importance of patient heterogeneity where different arms of a protocol can be effective on different subsets of patients.

The conclusion must be, however, that the disease, acute leukemia, remains far from totally cured and continuing advances can and will be made through the study and application of results from experimental leukemia models.

ACKNOWLEDGEMENTS

The research for and preparation of this Chapter was supported by PHS grant number CA 34144 awarded by the National Cancer Institute, DHHS; and by the Wayne State University Ben Kasle Trust for Cancer Research.

REFERENCES

1. Frei E: Intramural therapeutic research at the National Cancer Institute, Department of Medicine: 1955-1965. Cancer Treat. Rep. 68:21-30, 1984.
2. Baltimore D: Viral RNA-dependent DNA polymerase. Nature 226:1209-1211, 1970.
3. Experimental Leukemia. Marvin Rich (ed) Appleton-Century-Crofts, New York, 1968.
4. Gallo RC: Growth of human normal and leukemic T cells: T-cell growth factor (TCGF) and the isolation of a new class of RNA tumor viruses (HTLV). Blood Cells 7:313-329, 1981.
5. Reyes P, Hall TC: Synthesis of 5-fluorouridine 5'-phosphate by a pyrimidine phosphoribosyltransferase of mammalian origin - 11. Correlation between the tumor levels of the enzyme and the 5-fluorouracil-promoted increase in survival of tumor-bearing mice. Biochem. Pharmacol. 58:2587-2590, 1969.
6. Kohn KW, Ewig RAG, Erickson LC, Zwelling LA: Measurement of strand breaks and cross-links by alkaline elution in DNA repair. Vol. 1, Part B , Marcel Dekker, Inc., New York, 1981, pp. 379-401.
7. Zubrod CG: Origins and development of chemotherapy research at the National Cancer Institute. Cancer Chem. Rep. 68:9-19, 1984.
8. Venditti JM: Preclinical drug development: Rationale and methods. Sem. Oncol. 8:349-361, 1981.
9. Goldenberg GT, Begleiter A: Membrane transport of alkylating agents. Pharmacol. Therap. 8:237-274, 1979.
10. Kessel D, Wodinsky I: Thymidine kinase as a determinant of the response to 5-Fluoro-2'-deoxyuridine in transplantable murine leukemias. Molec. Pharmacol. 6:251-254, 1970.
11. Alt FW, Kellems RE, Bertino JR, Schimke RT: Selective multiplication of dihydrofolate reductase genes in methotrexate-resistant variants of cultured murine cells. J. Biol. Chem. 253:1357-1370, 1978.
12. Zwelling LA, Kohn KW: Mechanism of action of cis-dichlorodiammine-platinum (11). Cancer Treat. Rep. 63: 1439-1444, 1979.

13. Yamamoto KR, Stampfer MR, Tomkins GM: Receptors from glucocorticoid-sensitive lymphoma cells and two classes of insensitive clones: Physical and DNA-binding properties. Proc. Nat. Acad. Sc. 71:3901-3905, 1974.
14. Homo-Delarche F: Glucocorticoid receptors and steroid sensitivity in normal and neoplastic human lymphoid cells: A review. Cancer Res. 44:431-437, 1984.
15. Gehring U, Tomkins GM: A new mechanism for steroid unresponsiveness: Loss of nuclear binding activity of a steroid hormone receptor. Cell 3:301-306, 1974.
16. Braunschweiger P, Schiffer LM: Effect of Methylprednisolone on the cell kinetic response of C3H/HeJ mammary tumors to cyclophosphamide and adriamycin. Cancer Res. 39:3812-3815, 1979.
17. Goldin A, Mantel N, Greenhouse SW, Venditti JM, Humphreys SR: Factors influencing the specificity of action of an antileukemic agent (aminopterin). Time of treatment and dosage schedule. J. Natl. Cancer Inst. 14:311-314, 1954.
18. Goldin A, Venditti JM, Humphreys SR, Mantel N: Modification of treatment schedules in the management of advanced mouse leukemia with amethopterin. J. Natl. Cancer Inst. 17:203-212, 1956.
19. Condit PT, Eliel LP: Effects of large infrequent doses of a-methopterin on acute leukemia in children. J.A.M.A. 172:105-107, 1960.
20. Henderson ES: Acute lymphocytic leukemia. In: Leukemia, Gung FW, Henderson ES (eds), Grune and Stratton, New York, 1983, pp. 575-625.
21. Venditti JM: Treatment schedule dependency of experimentally active antileukemic (L1210) drugs. Cancer Chemother. Reports 2:Pt 3:35-59, 1971.
22. Goldin A, Venditti JM, Humphreys SR, Mantel N: Influence of the concentration of leukemic inoculum on the effectiveness of treatment. Science 123:840, 1956.
23. Puck TT, Marcus PI: Action of x-rays on mammalian cells. J. Expt. Med. 103:653-666, 1956.
24. Hewitt HB, Wilson CW: A survival curve for mammalian leukemia cells irradiated _in vivo_ (Implications for the treatment of mouse leukemia by whole body irradiation). Brit. J. Cancer 12:69-75, 1959.
25. Berry RJ: A comparison of effects of some chemotherapeutic agents and those of x-rays on the reproductive capacity of mammalian cells. Nature 203:1150-1153, 1964.
26. Bruce WR, Meeker BE, Valeriote FA: Comparison of the sensitivity of normal hematopoietic and transplanted lymphoma colony-forming cells to chemotherapeutic agents administered _in vivo_. J. Natl. Cancer Inst. 37:233-245, 1966.
27. Till JE, McCulloch EA: A direct measurement of the radiation sensitivity of normal mouse bone marrow cells. Radiat. Res. 14:213-222, 1965.

28. Skipper HE, Schabel FM Jr, Wilcox WS: Experimental evaluation of potential anticancer agents. XIII. On the criteria and kinetics associated with "curability" of experimental leukemia. Cancer Chem. Rep. 35:3-111, 1964.
29. Frei E, Canellos GP: Dose: A critical factor in cancer chemotherapy. Amer. J. Med. 69:585-594, 1980.
30. Kaplan HS: Evidence for tumoricidal dose level in the radiotherapy of Hodgkin's disease. Cancer Res. 26:1221-1224, 1966.
31. Pinkel D, Hernandez K, Borello L et al: Drug dosage and remission duration in childhood lymphocytic leukemia. Cancer 27:247-256, 1971.
32. Frei E, Freireich EJ: Progress and perspectives in the chemotherapy of acute leukemia. Adv. in Chemother. 2:269-298, 1965.
33. Skipper HE, Schabel FM Jr, Wilson WS: Experimental evaluation of potential anticancer agents. XXI. Scheduling of arabinosylsytosine to take advantage of its S-phase specificity against leukemia cells. Cancer Chem. Rep. 51:125-165, 1967.
34. Valeriote F: Cellular aspects of the action of cytosine arabinoside. Med. Ped. Oncol. Supp. 1:5-26, 1982.
35. Frei E, Bickers JN, Hewlett JS, Lane M, Leary MV, Talley, RW: Dose schedule and antitumor studies of arabinosyl cytosine (NSC 63878). Cancer Res. 29:1325-1332, 1969.
36. Furth J, Kahn MC, Breedis C: The transmission of leukemia of mice with a single cell. Amer. J. Cancer 31:276-282, 1937.
37. Cloning of Human Tumor Stem Cells. In: Prog. Clin. Biol. Res., Salmon SE (ed), Alan R. Liss, NY, 1980, Vol. 48.
38. McCulloch EA: Stem cells in normal and leukemic hemopoiesis. Blood 62:1-13, 1983.
39. Park CH, Bergsagel DE, McCulloch EA: Mouse myeloma tumor stem cells: A primary cell culture assay. J. Natl. Cancer Inst. 46:411-422, 1971.
40. Park CH, Bergsagel DE, McCulloch EA: Ascorbic acid: A culture requirement for colony formation by mouse plasmacytoma cell. Science 174:720-722, 1971.
41. Hamburger A, Salmon S: Primary bioassay of human myeloma stem cells. J. Clin. Invest. 60:846-854, 1977.
42. Buick RN, Minden MD, McCulloch EA: Self-renewal in culture of proliferating blast progenitor cells in acute myeloblastic leukemia. Blood 54:95-104, 1979.
43. Priesler HD: Prediction of response to chemotherapy in acute myelocytic leukemia. Blood 56:361-367, 1980.
44. Lin H, Bruce WR: A cellular approach to the chemotherapy of spontaneous leukemia of AKR mice. Ser. Hematol. 5:73-88, 1972.
45. Valeriote F, Lynch R, Berger NA, White E, Coulter D: Growth characteristics of MOPC-315 plasmacytoma and response to anti-cancer agents. J. Natl. Cancer Inst. 66:1083-1088, 1981.

46. Bush RS, Bruce WR: The radiation sensitivity of transplanted murine lymphoma cells as determined by the spleen colony method. Radiat. Res. 21:612-621, 1964.
47. Fertil B, Malise E-P: Inherent cellular radiosensitivity as a basic concept for human tumor radiotherapy. Int. J. Rad. Oncol. Biol. Phys. 7:621-629, 1981.
48. Weichselbaum RR, Nove J, Little JB: X-ray sensitivity of fifty-three human diploid fibroblast cell strains from patients with characterized genetic disorders. Cancer Res. 40:920-925, 1980.
49. Weichselbaum RR, Nove J, Little JB: X-ray sensitivity of human tumor cells _in vitro_. Int. J. Rad. Oncol. Biol. Phys. 6:437-440, 1980.
50. Sinclair WK: X-ray-induced heritable damage (small-colony formation) in cultured mammalian cells. Radiat. Res. 21: 584-611, 1964.
51. Elkind MM, Whitmore GF: The radiobiology of cultured mammalian cells. Gordon and Breach, New York, 1967.
52. Valeriote F, Tolen S: Protection and potentiation of nitrogen mustard cytotoxicity by WR-2721. Cancer Res. 42:4330-4331, 1982.
53. Mulcahy RT, Siemann DW: _In vivo_ chemosensitization by misonidazole in sensitive and resistant tumor lines. Cancer Res. 43:4709-4713, 1983.
54. Flentje M, Flentje D, Sapareto SA: Differential effect of hyperthermia on murine bone marrow NCFU and AKR- and L1210-leukemia stem cells. Cancer Res. 44:1761-1766, 1984.
55. Skipper HE, Chapman JB, Bell M: The anti-leukemic action of combinations of certain known anti-leukemic agents. Cancer Res. 11:109-112,1951.
56. Law LW: Effects of combinations of antileukemic agents on an acute lymphocytic leukemia of mice. Cancer Res. 12: 871-878, 1952.
57. Goldin A, Greenspan EM, Schoenbach EB: Studies on the mechanism of action of chemotherapeutic agents in cancer. VI. Synergistic (additive) action of drugs on a transplantable leukemia in mice. Cancer 5:153-160, 1952.
58. Goldin A, Venditti JM, Humphreys SR, Dennis D, Mantel N, Greenhouse SW: An investigation into the synergistic antileukemic action of amethopterin and 6-mercaptopurine in mice. J. Natl. Cancer Inst. 16:129-138, 1955.
59. Schabel FM Jr, Laster WR Jr, Trader M, Corbett TH, Griswold DP Jr: Combination chemotherapy with nitrosoureas plus other anticancer drugs against animal tumors. In: Nitrosoureas - Current Status and New Developments. Prestayko AW, Crooke ST, Baker LH, Carter SK, Schein PS (eds), Academic Press, New York, 1981, pp. 9-26.
60. Edelstein M, Vietti T, Valeriote F: Schedule-dependent synergism for the combination of 1-B-D-arabinofuranosylcytosine and daunorubicin. Cancer Res. 34:293-297, 1974.

61. Razek A, Vietti T, Valeriote F: Optimum time sequence for the administration of vincristine and cyclophosphamide in vivo. Cancer Res. 34:1875-1861, 1974.
62. Valeriote FA, Bruce WR, Meeker BE: Synergistic action of cyclophosphamide and 1,3-bis(2-chloroethyl)-1-nitrosourea on a transplanted murine lymphoma. J. Natl. Cancer Inst. 40:935-944, 1968.
63. Edelstein M, Vietti T, Valeriote F. The enhanced cytotoxicity of combinations of 1-B-D-arabinofuranosylcytosine and methotrexate. Cancer Res. 35:1555-1558, 1975.
64. Van Putten LM, Keizer HJ, Mulder JH: Perspectives in cancer research. Synchronization in tumor chemotherapy. Europ. J. Cancer 12:79-85, 1976.
65. Clarkson BD: Acute myelocytic leukemia in adults. Cancer 30:1572-1582, 1972.
66. Bryan JH, Henderson ES, Levinthal BG: Cytosine arabinoside and 6-thioguanine in refractory acute lymphocytic leukemia. Cancer 33:539-544, 1974.
67. Klein HO, Adler D, Doering M, Klein PJ, Lennartz KJ: Investigations on pharmacologic induction of partial synchronization of tumor cell proliferation: Its relevance for cytostatic therapy. Cancer Treat. Rep. 60:1959-1979, 1976.
68. Schabel FM Jr: The use of tumor growth kinetics in planning "curative" chemotherapy of advanced solid tumors. Cancer Res. 29:2384-2389, 1969.
69. Vincent PC: Kinetics of leukemia and control of cell division and replication. In: Leukemia, Gung FW, Henderson ES (eds), Grune and Stratton, New York, 1983, pp. 77-117.
70. Rosen PJ, Perry S, Schabel FM Jr: Proliferative capacity of leukemic cells in AKR leukemia. J. Natl. Cancer Inst. 45:1169-1178, 1970.
71. Vaughan WP, Karp JE, Burke PJ: Long chemotherapy-free remissions after single cycle timed-sequential chemotherapy for acute myelocytic leukemia. Cancer 45:859-865, 1980.
72. Burke PJ, Vaughan WP, Karp JE: A rationale for sequential high-dose chemotherapy of leukemia timed to coincide with induced tumor proliferation. Blood 55:960-968, 1980.
73. Goldin A, Venditti JM, Humphreys SR, Dennis D, Mantel N, Greenhouse, SW: Factors influencing the specificity of action of an antileukemic agent (aminopterin). Multiple treatment schedules plus delayed administration of citovorum factor. Cancer Res. 15:57-61, 1955.
74. Santelli G, Valeriote F: In vivo enhancement of 5-fluorouracil cytotoxicity to AKR leukemia cells by thymidine in mice. J. Natl. Cancer Inst. 61:843-847, 1978.
75. Santelli G, Valeriote F: In vivo potentiation of 5-fluorouracil cytotoxicity against AKR leukemia by purines, pyrimidines and their nucleosides and deoxynucleosides. J. Natl. Cancer Inst. 64:69-72, 1980.

76. Cadman E, Heimer R, Davis L: Enhanced 5-fluorouracil nucleotide formation after methotrexate administration: explanation for drug synergism. Science 205:1135-1137, 1979.

77. Moore EW, Thomas LB, Shaw RK, Freireich EJ: The central nervous system in acute leukemia. Arch. Internal Med. 105:141-158, 1960.

78. Nies BA, Bodey GP, Thomas LB, Brecher G, Freireich EJ: The persistence of extramedullary leukemia infiltrates during bone marrow remission of acute leukemia. Blood 26:133-141, 1965.

79. Aur RJA, Simone J, Hustu HO, Walters T, Borella L, Pratt C, Pinkel D: Central nervous system therapy and combination chemotherapy of childhood lymphocytic leukemia. Blood 37:272-281, 1971.

80. Skipper HE, Schabel FM Jr, Trader MW, Thomson JR: Experimental evaluation of potential anticancer agents. VI. Anatomical distribution of leukemic cells and failure of chemotherapy. Cancer Res. 21:1154-1164, 1961.

81. Schabel FM Jr, Johnston TP, McCaleb GS, Montgomery JA, Laster WR, Skipper HE: Experimental evaluation of potential anticancer agents VIII. Effects of certain nitrosoureas on intracerebral L1210 leukemia. Cancer Res. 23: 725-733, 1963.

82. Johnson RE: An experimental therapeutic approach to L1210 leukemia in mice: Combined chemotherapy and central nervous system irradiation. J. Natl. Cancer Inst. 32: 1333-1341, 1964.

83. Mauer AM: Current therapy for acute lymphocytic leukemia: Is it rational? Blood Cells 8:553-560, 1982.

84. Lynch RG, Medoff G, Valeriote F: A murine model for central nervous system leukemia and its possible relevance to human leukemia. J. Natl. Cancer Inst. 55:611-617, 1975.

85. Till JE, McCulloch EA: A direct measurement of the radiation sensitivity of normal mouse bone marrow cells. Radiat. Res. 14:213-222, 1961.

86. Valeriote F, van Putten L: Proliferation-dependent cytotoxicity of anticancer agents: A review. Cancer Res. 35:2619-2630, 1975.

87. Valeriote FA, Bruce WR: Comparison of the sensitivity of hematopoietic colony-forming cells in different proliferative states to vinblastine. J. Natl. Cancer Inst. 38: 393-399, 1967.

88. Bradley TR, Metcalf D: The growth of mouse bone marrow cells _in vitro_. Aust. J. Exp. Biol. Med. Sci. 44:287-300, 1966.

89. Sachs L: Control of growth and normal differentiation in leukemic cells: Regulation of the developmental programs and restoration of the normal phenotype in myeloid leukemia. J. Cell Physiol. Supp. 1:151-164, 1982.

90. Sachs L: Regulation of normal cell differentiation and malignancy in myeloid leukemia. In: Differentiation of Normal and Neoplastic Hematopoietic Cells. Book A, Clarkson B, Marks PA, Till JE (eds), Cold Spring Harbor Laboratory, 1978, pp. 411-423.
91. Bloch A: Induced cell differentiation in cancer therapy. Cancer Treat. Rep. 68:199-205, 1984.
92. Castaigne S, Daniel MT, Lilly H, Horait P, Degos L: Does treatment with Ara-C in low dosage cause differentiation of leukemic cells. Blood 62:85-86, 1983.
93. Broxmeyer HE, Smithyman A, Eger RR et al: Identification of lactoferrin as the granulocyte-derived inhibitor of colony-stimulating activity production. J. Exp. Med. 148:1052-1067, 1978.
94. Wiernik PH: Acute leukemias of adults. In: Cancer. Principles and Practice of Oncology. DeVita VT Jr, Hellman S, Rosenberg SA (eds), J.B. Lippincott, Philadelphia, 1982, pp. 1402-1426,
95. Dexter TM: Stromal cell associated hemopoiesis. J. Cell Physiol. Supp. 1:87-94, 1982.
96. Glascow G, Beetham KL, Mill WB: Dose rate effects on the survival of normal hematopoietic stem cells of BALB/C mice. Intl. J. Rad. Oncol. Biol. Phys. 9:557-563, 1983.
97. Lorenz E, Uphoff D, Reid TR, Skelton E: Modification of irradiation injury in mice and guinea pigs by bone marrow injections. J. Natl. Cancer Inst. 12:197-201, 1951.
98. Thomas ED, Storb R, Clift RA et al: Bone marrow transplantation. New Eng. J. Med. 292:832-843, 1975.
99. Mathe G: Immunotherapie active de la Llucemie L1210 applique apres la greffe tumorale. Rev. Franc. Etudes Clin. et Biol. 13:881-883, 1968.
100. Mathe G, Amiel JL, Schwarzenberg L, Schneider M, Cattan, A Schlumberger JR, Hayat M, de Vassal F: Active immunotherapy for acute lymphoblastic leukemia. Lancet i:697-699, 1969.
101. Amiel J-L: Immunotherapie active non specifique par le B.C.G. de la leucemie virale E G_2 chez des receveurs isogeniques. Rev. Franc. Etudes Clin. et Biol. 12:912-914, 1967.
102. Amiel JL, Berardet M: An experimental model of active immunotherapy preceded by cytoreductive chemotherapy. Europ. J. Cancer 6:557-559, 1970.
103. Valeriote F, Lynch R, Medoff G, Tolen S, Dieckman J: Growth and rejection of leukemia cells in individual mice after combined treatment with amphotericin B and 1,3-bis(2-chloroethyl)-1-nitrosourea. J. Natl. Cancer Inst. 61:399-402, 1978.
104. Medoff G, Valeriote F, Ryan J, Tolen S: Response of transplanted AKR leukemia to combination therapy with amphotericin B and 1,3-bis(2-chloroethyl)-1-nitrosourea: dose and schedule dependency. J. Nat. Cancer Inst. 58: 949-953, 1977.

105. Ducos R, Valeriote F: Quantitation of the immune rejection of allotransplanted AKR leukemia cells. Transplantation 21:279-281, 1976.
106. Lynch RG, Rohrer JW, Odermatt B, Gebel HM, Autry JR, Hoover RG: Immunoregulation of murine myeloma cell growth and differentiation: A monoclonal model of B cell differentiation. Immunol. Rev. 48:45-80, 1979.
107. Olsson L, Mathe G: Antigenic heterogeneity of leukemia. Blood Cells 7:281-286, 1981.
108. Dexter DL, Kowalski HM, Blazar BA et al: Heterogeneity of tumor cells from a single mouse mammary tumor. Cancer Res. 38:3174-3181, 1978.
109. Rosenberg SA: Adoptive immunotherapy of cancer: Accomplishments and prospects. Cancer Treat. Rep. 68:233-255, 1984.
110. Curt GA, Clendeninn NJ, Chabner BA: Drug resistance in Cancer. Cancer Treat. Rep. 68:87-99, 1984.
111. Kessel D, Hall TC, Roberts D, Wodinsky I: Uptake as a determinant of methotrexate response in mouse leukemias. Science 150:752-754, 1965.
112. Inaba M, Johnson RK: Uptake and retention of adriamycin and daunorubicin by sensitive and anthracycline-resistant sublines of P388 leukemia. Biochem. Pharmacol. 27:2123-2130, 1978.
113. Suzukake K, Petro BJ, Vistica DT: Reduction in glutathione content of L-Pam-resistant L1210 cells confer drug sensitivity. Biochem. Pharmacol. 32:121-124, 1982.
114. Tsuruo T, Iida H, Nojiri M, Tsukagoshi S, Sakurai Y: Circumvention of vincristine and adriamycin resistance <u>in vitro</u> and <u>in vivo</u> by calcium influx blockers. Cancer Res. 43:2905-2910, 1983.
115. Valeriote F, Medoff G, Dieckman J: Potentiation of anticancer agent cytotoxicity against sensitive and resistant AKR leukemia by amphotericin B. Cancer Res. 39:2041-2045, 1979.
116. Vainchenker W, Testa U, Guichard J, Titeux M, Breton-Gorius J: Heterogeneity in the cellular commitment of a human leukemic cell line: K562. Blood Cells 7:357-375, 1981.

3

CLINICAL LABORATORY METHODS USED FOR THE CLASSIFICATION OF ACUTE LEUKEMIA

Margarita Palutke, M.D.

Until a few years ago morphologic examination and cytochemical techniques were the only readily available tools in characterizing acute leukemias. With advances in chemotherapy accurate identification of the leukemic cell types has become essential. The clinical laboratory can now provide a great variety of additional tests resulting in the precise definition of many clinicopathological entities. These tests utilize immunological, biochemical and cytogenetic methods, and flow cytometric analysis of DNA content.

1. DIAGNOSTIC PROCEDURES

1.1 Morphology and cytochemistry

To standardize morphologic classification of acute leukemias, a cooperative French-American-British (FAB) group in 1976 established criteria for six myeloblastic (M1 - M6) and three lymphoblastic variants (L1 - L3) of acute leukemia (FAB classification, Table 1) (1). The morphologic characteristics observed in blood and bone marrow were supplemented by a few cytochemical reactions such as myeloperoxidase, Sudan black B, and non-specific esterase reactions. Since the identification of lymphoblastic leukemias, as a rule, was not aided by cytochemical staining, a more detailed morphologic evaluation system was established in 1981, based on two major criteria: nuclear to cytoplasmic ratio and nucleolar features, and two minor criteria: nuclear shape and cell size (2).

The importance of recognizing M3 and especially the microgranular variant of M3 (3,4) lies in the fact that both are frequently accompanied by intravascular coagulopathies which require prompt and aggressive therapy. The microgranular variant may be confused with acute monocytic leukemia unless cytochemical stains, such as myeloperoxidase, are performed. With these stains numerous Auer rods and secondary granules become very apparent in the microgranular variant of M3.

TABLE 1

FRENCH-AMERICAN-BRITISH (FAB) CLASSIFICATION

M1	myeloblastic leukemia without maturation
M2	myeloblastic leukemia with evidence of maturation
M3	hypergranular progranulocytic leukemia, including the micrognanular variant
M4	myelomonocytic leukemia
M5	monocytic leukemia a. poorly differentiated b. differentiated
M6	erythroleukemia
L1	acute lymphoblastic leukemia, predominantly of small cell size
L2	acute lymphoblastic leukemia, predominantly of large cell size
L3	Burkitt-type leukemia

The value of the FAB classification has been questioned. Concordance rates between observers can be less than 40% to 60%

(5-7). Better concordance rates are obtained when experienced hematomorphologists perform the examination which includes standardized cytochemical techniques (5,7).

The clinical significance of the FAB classification has also been questioned. No prognostic significance of distinguishing M1, M2 and M4 has been demonstrated by some (6,9). Others suggest that patients whose disease was categorized as M1, M5a or M6 appeared to do less well than patients with M2, M3, M4 or M5b disease (10,11). The best prognostic parameter was the presence of Auer rods. Complete remission was achieved in 68% of patients whose leukemic cells had Auer rods and in only 40% of those whose cells lacked Auer rods.

In the lymphoid categories, L2 and L3 generally have a poorer prognosis than L1. However, L2 more frequently occurs in adults whose prognosis with all acute leukemias is worse than it is in children. Unfortunately, the L1 and L2 variants do not correspond to immunologic phenotypes which define distinct clinicopathological entities.

Although the value of the FAB classification is disputed, recent progress in cytogenetic phenotyping of various leukemias may make it possible to correlate FAB categories (12) with specific clinicopathological entities. At the present time, the FAB classification provides a common language for experts in the field.

Table 2 is a list of cytochemical reactions frequently used in our laboratory for the diagnosis of acute leukemia. In evaluating the reactions, several characteristics or features are noted and described: intensity of staining, distribution of staining (dispersed or localized; in fine granules or blocklike), and the cytoplasmic background of the cells (clear or diffusely colored).

Cells of acute myeloblastic leukemia generally stain with myeloperoxidase and/or Sudan black B and/or naphthol AS-D chloroacetate esterase. Cells of acute monocytic leukemia generally stain with alpha-naphthyl acetate and butyrate (non-specific esterase). Sodium fluoride will inhibit these reactions in monoblasts. T cell lymphoblastic leukemia will usually have localized staining in the Golgi region with acid phosphatase, whereas most of the other leukemias have a diffuse granular positivity. A block-like, coarse PAS positivity is most frequently associated with acute lymphoblastic leukemia, although we have on rare occasions observed it in acute monocytic leukemia.

TABLE 2

FREQUENTLY USED CYTOCHEMICAL REACTIONS FOR IDENTIFICATION OF ACUTE LEUKEMIAS

Myeloperoxidase
Sudan Black B
Naphthol AS-D Chloroacetate Esterase
Alpha-Naphthyl Acetate
Alpha-Naphthyl Acetate with Sodium Fluoride (NaF)
Alpha-Naphthyl Butyrate
Acid Phosphatase
Periodic Acid-Schiff

For more detailed descriptions of the morphological characteristics of the various acute leukemias in the FAB classification and their cytochemical reactions, a recent review article by Bell et al (8) is recommended.

1.2 Immunology

As recently as the 1970's immunologic testing was restricted to a few procedures which helped to define several different subtypes of acute lymphocytic leukemia. Except for L3 which was found to have monoclonal surface immunoglobulin and thus could be classified as a B cell malignancy (13), the immunologic typing did not correspond to the FAB classification of acute lymphocytic leukemia (ALL) (14). The presence of lymphoblasts which cause spontaneous sheep erythrocyte rosette (E rosette) formation characterizes a subtype of ALL with a distinct clinicopathological picture and a poor prognosis (15). However, such leukemias could fall into either the L1 or L2 category. Another subtype of ALL, the pre-B cell leukemia, was identified as consisting of blasts that contained intracytoplasmic mu chains without light chains or surface immunoglobulin (16). Here also, the FAB classification fails since such leukemias may be classified as either L1 or L2.

In the last few years, numerous monoclonal antisera to differentiation antigens of the hematopoietic cell lines have been used to classify acute leukemia (17). For practical purposes, the diagnostically most helpful antisera have been those directed at the lymphocytic differentiation antigens.

Table 3 illustrates the most helpful, commercially available monoclonal antisera. Antisera to antigens of cells of monocytic or myeloid lineage are only occasionally useful because of cross-reactivity with each other and with null cells.

1.3 Chemistry

Terminal deoxynucleotidyl transferase (TdT) is an enzyme which catalyzes the polymerization of deoxyribonucleotides on the 3'-OH end of polydeoxyribonucleotides. Until recently it was regarded as a rather specific enzyme found in thymic cells (18). Its detection in lymphoblasts of a child with acute lymphoblastic leukemia initially suggested that this enzyme was found in leukemic lymphoblasts derived from the thymic cell population (19,20). However, recently, this enzyme has been found in cells of null ALL as well as T-ALL, in lymphoblastic lymphoma, in chronic myelogenous leukemia in blast crisis (21), in pre-B cell ALL (22), and occasionally in acute myeloblastic leukemia (21). Despite the apparently ubiquitous presence of this enzyme, it is a diagnostic aid when combined with the immunologic phenotypes of the acute leukemias (Table 3).

TABLE 3

IMMUNOLOGIC PHENOTYPES OF ACUTE LEUKEMIA

MONOCLONAL ANTIBODY	TYPES OF ACUTE LEUKEMIA					
	COMMON ALL*	T ALL	B ALL	PRE-B ALL	NULL ALL	ANLL**
Anti-CALLA	+***	-	-	+	-	-
Anti-B	-	-	+	+	-	-
Anti-T11 (anti RBC sheep receptor antibody)	-	+	-	-	-	-
Anti-Ia	+	-	+	+	+ or -	+ or -
TdT	+	+	-	+	+	usually -

*ALL = acute lymphocytic leukemia.
**ANLL = acute non-lymphocytic leukemia.
***+ and - refer to presence or absence of reactivity of leukemic cells with respective antibody.

This test should be interpreted, with caution, when the leukemic cells represent a minor population in a bone marrow sample. In normal bone marrow, 2 to 20% of cells thought to be hematogones, contain TdT (23).

Lysozyme (muramidase) determination in urine or serum may be of great help in the diagnosis of monocytic or myelomonocytic leukemia when cytochemical reactions are not diagnostic, elevated levels frequently being present in such cases.

1.4 Cytogenetics

Improved high resolution banding techniques for studying human chromosomes provide evidence that chromosomal defects are present in most malignancies (12). In many, the defects are consistent. In acute leukemias, specific chromosomal defects have been reported to correlate with some of the FAB categories (12). In M3 (hypergranular progranulocytic leukemia) the chromosomal defect t(15;17) is thought to be characteristic of this leukemia. Other cytogenetic abnormalities in acute leukemias are: t(9;22) in M1; t(8;21) in M2; inv(16) in M4; t(9;11) in M4 and M5; del 5q, del 7q, +8 in M1, M2, M4, M5 and M6; t(9;22) in L1 and L2; t(4;11) in L2; and t(8;14) in L3.

1.5 DNA content analysis

By means of flow cytometry the DNA content of cell nuclei can be measured after staining with DNA-binding fluorochromes such as propidium iodide, ethidium bromide, mithramycin, and acridine orange. Aneuploidy can be detected by comparing DNA content of leukemic nuclei in G1 phase to those of normal control leukocytes. The percentage of cells in S phase may give an indication of the aggressiveness of the malignancy. A prognostic significance of the chromosome number in acute lymphoblastic leukemia in children was demonstrated by several investigators using both flow cytometry and cytogenetics (24-26). A near haploid number of chromosomes was found to predict a poor prognosis (24), whereas a hyperdiploid number suggested a better outlook than a diploid number (26). High percentages of S phase cells indicated a more aggressive tumor (26).

Flow cytometric techniques detect aneuploidy much faster than cytogenetic studies. However, these techniques are still limited because at least two chromosomes in excess of, or less than, the normal number are needed to be detectable. Also, the technique does not, as yet, provide identification of specific chromosomal abnormalities.

2. CONCLUSION

Many clinical laboratories in large medical centers are now equipped to provide multiparameter diagnostic testing designed to accurately define the cell type of leukemic blasts. This is necessary to identify specific clinicopathological entities which can be treated with appropriate therapeutic regimens.

REFERENCES

1. Bennett JM, Catovsky D, Daniel MT, Flandrin G, Galton DAG, Gralnick HR, Sultan C: Proposals for the classification of the acute leukaemias. Br. J. Haematol. 33:451-458, 1976.
2. Bennett JM, Catovsky D, Daniel MT, Flandrin G, Galton DAG, Gralnick HR, Sultan C: The morphological classification of acute lymphoblastic leukemia: Concordance among observers and clinical correlations. Br. J. Haematol. 47:553-561, 1981.
3. Savage RA, Hoffman GC, Lucas FV: Morphology and cytochemistry of microgranular acute promyelocytic leukemia (M3m). Am. J. Clin. Pathol. 75:548-552, 1981.
4. Golomb HM, Rowley JD, Vardiman JW, Testa JR, Butler A: "Microgranular" acute promyelocytic leukemia: A distinct clinical, ultrastructural, and cytogenetic entity. Blood 55:253-259, 1980.
5. Dick FR, Armitage JO, Burns CP: Diagnostic concurrence in the subclassification of adult acute leukemia using French-American-British criteria. Cancer 49:916-920, 1982.
6. Bennett JM, Begg CB: Eastern Cooperative Oncology Group study of the cytochemistry of adult acute myeloid leukemia by correlation of subtypes with response and survival. Cancer Res. 41:4833-4837, 1981.
7. Head DR, Cerezo L, Savage RA, Craven CM, Bickers JN, Hartsock R, Hosty TA, Saiki JH, Wilson HE, Morrison FS, Coltman CA, Hutton JJ: Institutional performance in application of the FAB classification of acute leukemia: The Southwest Oncology Group experience. Cancer (In press).
8. Bell A, Hippel T, Goodman H: Use of cytochemistry and FAB classification in leukemia and other pathological states. Focus 47:437-471, 1981.
9. Bozdach MJ, Kurowski KS, Brynildson SM, Schilling RF: Survival in adult acute leukemia: Correlation with morphology, age and cytogenetics. Blood 85(Suppl):135a, 1981.
10. Mertelsmann R, Thaler HT, To L, Gee TS, McKenzie S, Schauer P, Friedman A, Arlin Z, Cirrincione C, Clarkson B: Morphological classification, response to therapy, and survival in 263 adult patients with acute non-lymphoblastic leukemia. Blood 56:773-781, 1980.

11. Sultan C, Deregnaucourt J, Ko YW, Imbert M, D'Agar MFR, Gouault-Heilmann M, Brun B: Distribution of 250 cases of acute myeloid leukemia (AML) according to the FAB classification and response to therapy. Br. J. Haematol. 47:545-551, 1981.
12. Yunis JJ: The chromosomal basis of human neoplasia. Science 221:227-236, 1983.
13. Flandrin G, Brouet JC, Daniel MT, Preud'homme JL: Acute leukemia with Burkitt's tumor cells: A study of six cases with special reference to lymphocyte surface markers. Blood 45:183-188, 1975.
14. Palutke M, Tabaczka P: Cytochemical and immunological aspects of the acute lymphocytic leukemias (as related to FAB classification). Ann. Clin. Lab. Sci. 10:269-275, 1980.
15. Borella L, Sen L: E receptors on blasts from untreated acute lymphocytic leukemia (ALL): Comparison of temperature dependence of E rosettes formed by normal and leukemic lymphoid cells. J. Immunol. 114:187-190, 1975.
16. Vogler LB, Crist WM, Bockman DE, Pearl ER, Lawton AR, Cooper MD: Pre-B cell leukemia: A new phenotype of childhood lymphoblastic leukemia. N. Eng. J. Med. 298:872-878, 1978.
17. Foon KA, Schroff RW, Gale RP: Surface markers on leukemia and lymphoma cells: Recent advances. Blood 60:1-15, 1982.
18. Chang LMS: Development of terminal deoxynucleotidyl transferase activity in embryonic calf thymus gland. Biochem. Biophys. Res. Commun. 44:124-131, 1971.
19. McCaffrey R, Harrison TA, Parkman R, Baltimore D: Terminal deoxynucleotidyl transferase activity in human leukemic cells and in normal human thymocytes. N. Eng. J. Med. 292:775-780, 1975.
20. McCaffrey R, Smoler DF, Baltimore D: Terminal deoxynucleotidyl transferase in a case of childhood acute lymphoblastic leukemia. Proc. Natl. Acad. Sci. 70:521- 525, 1973.
21. Kung PC, Long JC, McCaffrey RP, Ratliff RL, Harrison TA, Baltimore D: Terminal deoxynucleotidyl transferase in the diagnosis of leukemia and malignant lymphoma. Am. J. Med. 64:788-794, 1978.
22. Brouet JC, Preud'homme JL, Penit C, Valensi F, Rouget P, Seligman M: Acute lymphoblastic leukemia with pre-B-cell characteristics. Blood 54:269-273, 1979.
23. Muehleck SD, McKenna RW, Gale PF, Brunning RD: Terminal deoxynucleotidyl transferase (TdT)-positive cells in bone marrow in the absence of hematologic malignancy. Am. J. Clin. Pathol. 79:277-283, 1983.
24. Brodeur GM, Williams DL, Look AT, Bowman WP, Kalwinsky DK: Near-haploid acute lymphoblastic leukemia: A unique subgroup with a poor prognosis? Blood 58:14-19, 1981.

25. Williams DL, Tsiatis A, Brodeur GM, Look AT, Melvin S, Bowman WP, Kalwinsky DK, Rivera G, Dahl GV: Prognostic importance of chromosome number in 136 untreated children with acute lymphoblastic leukemia. Blood 60:864-871, 1982.

26. Look AT, Melvin SL, Williams DL, Brodeur GM, Dahl GV, Kalwinsky DK, Murphy SB, Mauer AM: Aneuploidy and percentage of S-phase cells determined by flow cytometry correlated with cell phenotype in childhood acute leukemia. Blood 60:959-967, 1982.

4

HTLV-II AND HUMAN LEUKEMIA

William Wachsman, Judith C. Gasson, David W. Golde and Irvin S.Y. Chen

Human T-cell leukemia virus (HTLV) is a type C retrovirus associated with some adult T-cell leukemias and lymphomas (1-3). HTLV-associated leukemia/lymphoma is endemic in southwestern Japan (adult T-cell leukemia) and parts of the Caribbean and is seen sporadically throughout the world. Evidence for a causal relationship between HTLV and this distinct T-cell neoplasia is strong; however, the mechanism of HTLV-induced leukemogenesis is unknown.

The majority of HTLV isolates, termed HTLV-I, are identical by nucleic acid hybridization and immunologic cross-reactivity. We have studied a patient with a different disease phenotype who proved to harbor a related virus termed HTLV-II. This paper provides a summary of our current state of knowledge of HTLV-II.

1. IDENTIFICATION OF HTLV-II

In 1978 we reported that a T-lymphoblast line (Mo) had been established from primary culture of splenic tissue obtained from a patient with a rare T-cell variant hairy-cell leukemia (HCL) (4). Phenotypic characterization of the Mo cells revealed them to be mature helper/inducer T-cells (Table I) (4,5). The cell line produces a variety of lymphokines, some constitutively and others after exogenous stimulation (Table II) (6-8).

Following the discovery and isolation of HTLV-I from the HUT-102 cell line by Gallo and co-workers (1), a radioimmunoassay was established for the HTLV p24 core antigens. This radioimmunoassay demonstrated the presence of cross-reactive antigen in the Mo cells. Competitive radioimmunoassay showed that the Mo p24 antigen was immunologically distinct from that of HTLV-I. The Mo subtype of HTLV was therefore designated HTLV-II (9).

TABLE I: Mo T-CELL CHARACTERIZATION

Morphology - lymphoblast		
Cytochemistry -	tartrate-resistant acid phosphatase (TRAP)$^{+}$ fluoride-resistant nonspecific esterase^{+} β-glucuronidase^{+} terminal deoxynucleotidyl transferase (TdT)$^{-}$	
Karyotype - normal 46XY		
Immunologic markers -	positive:	Leu-1, Leu-3a, OKT-4, anti-Dr antibody, sheep red blood cell rosette formation
	negative:	Leu-2a, OKT-8, cytoplasmic immunoglobulin, surface immunoglobulin
Other - negative for Epstein-Barr virus		

TABLE II: LYMPHOKINES ELABORATED FROM Mo-T CELLS

Colony-stimulating factor (CSF)[a]
Erythroid-potentiating activity (EPA)[a]
Fibroblast growth factor[a]
Gamma interferon[b]
Macrophage-activating factor (MAF)[a]
Macrophage migration-inhibitory factor (MIF)[b]
Neutrophil migration-inhibition factor from T-lymphocytes (NIF-T)[a]

[a] Constitutive production

[b] Induction by mitogens or phorbol myristate

2. CLINICAL PERSPECTIVE

There is a striking contrast between the diseases associated with HTLV-I and HTLV-II. The former is found in patients with a highly aggressive, mature T-cell leukemia/lymphoma often associated with skin and bone lesions as well as hypercalcemia (10-12). The acute form carries a poor prognosis. By comparison, the patient Mo presented with mild constitutional symptoms, marked splenomegaly, and pancytopenia. After the diagnosis of hairy-cell leukemia was established, therapeutic splenectomy was performed. Subsequently, the symptoms and pancytopenia resolved, and he is alive and well more than eight years after diagnosis. There has been no evidence of progressive disease or hypercalcemia. Mo's chronic course is similar to that seen in both B-cell HCL and the T-cell variant of HCL (less than 2 percent of cases) (13). Hairy cells are still present in his peripheral blood (10-20 percent of circulating lymphocytes) and he continues to maintain a significant serum level of antibody to HTLV-II p24 core antigen. In addition, primary culture of the patient's peripheral blood obtained seven years post-splenectomy has resulted in the establishment of one T-cell line and two B-cell lines infected with HTLV-II (unpublished observation).

It is not understood why the clinical syndromes associated with HTLV-I and HTLV-II are so different, although it likely relates to differences in the molecular structure of the viruses (see below). Only a single patient with HTLV-II-associated disease has been identified, and detection of other patients with HTLV-II and further *in vitro* studies on HTLV comparative biology will be needed to answer this question.

3. MOLECULAR CLONING OF HTLV-II

To better define the biology of HTLV-II and compare it to HTLV-I we molecularly cloned the HTLV-II provirus (14). Due to low levels of virus produced by the Mo cells, viral cDNA clones were first isolated from a cDNA library prepared from mRNA of HTLV-II-infected Mo cells. The viral cDNA clones were then used to probe a lambda genomic library constructed from Mo DNA. Three distinct proviral clones were identified (Figure 1). The first, λH-6, was 8.8 kbp in length and was bounded at both ends by long terminal repeats (LTRs). This provirus represents the complete, replication-competent HTLV-II genome. The other two proviral clones isolated, λH-9 (6.5 kbp) and λH-2 (3.5 kbp), were similar at the 3' and 5' ends to λ H-6, but contained large internal deletions.

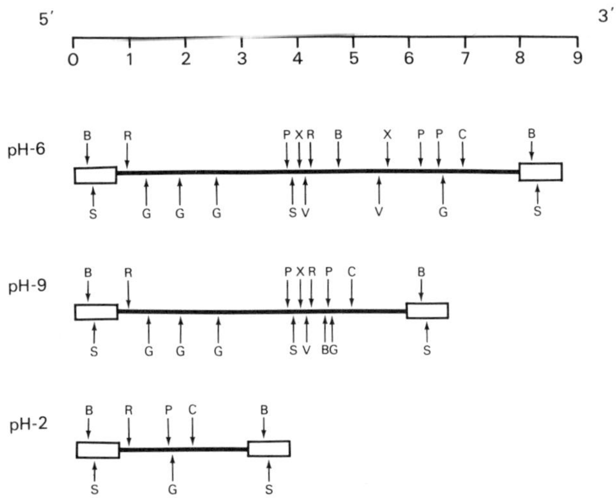

Figure 1: RESTRICTION MAPPING OF HTLV-II PROVIRUSES FROM LATE PASSAGE Mo

Cloned inserts representing the three HTLV-II proviruses are shown. The viral sequences including LTRs are represented by a solid bar flanked by two open boxes. Flanking human cellular sequences and the plasmid vector, pBR322, are not shown. The 5' and 3' ends of the genomes are indicated. The numbers marked above the genomes denote size in kbp. Sites of cleavage are represented for the following restriction enzymes: BamHI (B), SacI (S), EcoRI (R), BglII (G), PstI (P), XhoI (X), PvuII (V), and ClaI (C).

Using the method of Southern, no hybridization of HTLV-II probes with DNA from cells infected and transformed by HTLV-I was detected under standard conditions, indicating significant differences between the sequences of the two HTLV types. Our nucleic acid sequence analysis of the HTLV-II LTR confirmed the limited sequence homology between HTLV-I and HTLV-II (15,16). These data, in conjunction with the previously defined partial cross-reactivity of HTLV-I and -II p24, demonstrate that the two subtypes of HTLV are only distantly related.

4. BIOLOGICAL PROPERTIES OF HTLV-II

Similar to HTLV-I, co-culture of HTLV-II-infected cells with normal human peripheral blood leukocytes leads to transformation of the normal T lymphocytes as defined by their ability to proliferate indefinitely (17-20). Within two to four weeks after co-cultivating lethally irradiated Mo cells with normal leukocytes, newly infected cells are detected by an indirect immunofluorescence assay for p24 and p19 antigens (20). Southern hybridization using HTLV-II probes reveals the presence of the HTLV-II provirus in DNA from transformed cell lines. To show that the transformed cells were derived from the normal cells, female donors were used and karyotypic analysis of the transformants showed a normal female karyotype in contrast to the Mo cell, which carries a normal male karyotype. These HTLV-II transformants are phenotypically and cytochemically similar to the Mo cell line (see Table I), that is, mature helper/inducer T cells. The Mo cells produce a variety of lymphokines and the transformant cells also produce many of these same lymphokines (21).

Cellular transformation could also be accomplished using lethally irradiated transformant cells derived from co-cultivation with Mo (20). In addition, transformant cells can be used in co-cultivation to transmit HTLV-II and transform normal cells from the same donor. Thus, the capacity to infect and transform normal cells is not a unique feature of Mo cells, nor is it necessary that conditions for an HLA-induced mixed lymphocyte reaction be present in the co-cultivation system.

Another cell line was established from the peripheral blood of the patient Mo about two years after splenectomy (20). This lymphoblastoid cell line, Mo-B, is negative for T-cell markers, does not produce lymphokines, has surface membrane immunoglobulin, and harbors Epstein-Barr virus (EBV). Analysis of the Mo-B cells revealed the presence of the HTLV-II provirus and the expression of the p19 and p24 core antigens. Co-culture of lethally irradiated Mo-B cells with normal peripheral blood leukocytes resulted in the outgrowth of HTLV-II-infected T-cell transformants. Cells competent for productive infection by HTLV-II appear to be limited to some subsets of mature T cells and EBV-transformed B cells. This lymphotropic property of HTLV-II is discussed below.

5. HTLV-II AND LEUKEMOGENESIS

5.1 Functions of the LTR

During the replication of retroviruses, the virus must enter a target host cell, produce a DNA copy of the genome by reverse transcription, integrate into host cell DNA, and produce genomic RNA and subgenomic mRNA transcripts for the formation of progeny virions. The proviral LTR contains sequences responsible for regulating reverse transcription, proviral integration, and proviral transcription (22,23). Studies of the HTLV-II LTR were designed to investigate the function of the LTR in HTLV-associated leukemogenesis, specifically of lymphoid cells and transformation of T-lymphoid cells.

Comparison of the nucleic acid sequence of the LTR of HTLV-I and -II shows little overall homology (15,16); however, there are strong sequence similarities in areas of the LTR critical for its regulatory function (15). Sequence homologies are evident in regions of the LTR known to be important for viral transcription: the TATAA box, the cap site, and the polyadenylation signal. It is notable that the polyadenylation signal for both viruses is located in an unusual position for most eukaryotic genes, about 250 nucleotides further upstream from its normal location. In addition, a unique 21-base triple repeat upstream of the TATAA box in the U3 region is conserved in both types of HTLV. These sequences may be involved in proviral transcriptional control.

As mentioned above, we have not observed productive infection of nonlymphoid cells by HTLV-II. Epithelial B-lymphoid hybrid cells that were co-cultured with Mo have shown the presence of HTLV-II proviruses, but no production of virus (24). In order to test the transcriptional function of the HTLV-II LTR in lymphoid and nonlymphoid cells, we constructed a variety of recombinant genomes of the HTLV-II LTR with the selectable marker neo^R in transfection assays in both Mo cells and fibroblasts (143 cells were derived from a human osteosarcoma). The results demonstrated that the HTLV-II LTR did not function to promote transcription in the 143 fibroblast cell line, but functioned efficiently in the Mo cells (24). The mechanism of HTLV-II LTR transcriptional restriction in non-lymphoid cells is unknown. The location of the 21-base triple repeat upstream of the TATAA box in both HTLV-II and HTLV-I suggests that it may function as a tissue-specific transcriptional enhancer sequence (25).

5.2 Oncogenes and HTLV-II-induced transformation

Since HTLV transforms T lymphocytes *in vitro* it could be classified as an acutely transforming retrovirus. Yet, unlike most other highly oncogenic retroviruses, nether HTLV-I nor HTLV-II have sequences in their genomes with nucleic acid homology to normal cellular sequences (viral oncogenes). HTLV biologically behaves like an acutely transforming retrovirus, but structurally resembles a weakly oncogenic replication-competent retrovirus (26).

Some weakly oncogenic retroviruses, such as avian leukosis viruses or Moloney murine leukemia viruses, mediate malignant transformation via the integration into host cellular DNA in the vicinity of cellular oncogenes with subsequent transcriptional activation of these genes (27,28). We determined whether there were any common sites of HTLV integration in HTLV-II-transformed cells. A genomic library constructed from DNA of an HTLV-II transformant cell line was screened and nine clones representing at least 5 different integrated proviruses were characterized. Cellular sequences flanking the proviruses were subcloned and used as probes to screen DNA prepared from nine different HTLV-II transformant cell lines and the Mo cell line. No evidence for a common site of HTLV-II integration was found (unpublished observation). Similarly, the pattern for HTLV-I proviral integration appears to be random (29).

HTLV may carry sequences necessary for transformation, which do not have an identifiable cellular homologue. If so, such sequences are likely to be present in the so called pX region.

5.3 The pX region

The structure of HTLV proviruses is similar to that of other retroviruses. LTRs are located at the 5' and 3' ends and encompass the *gag*, *pol*, and *env* structural genes that encode the core proteins, reverse transcriptase, and envelope proteins, respectively. In addition, both subtypes of HTLV contain approximately 1.5 kbp of novel sequence at the 3' end, termed pX, whose function is unknown. From the sequence analysis of HTLV-I, four open reading frames were delineated that could potentially encode four proteins of molecular weights ranging from 10,000 to 27,000 daltons (30). Comparison of predicted HTLV-I and HTLV-II amino acid sequences, based on the known HTLV-I nucleic acid sequence and partial HTLV-II nucleic acid sequence, reveals about 70 percent homology in pX and about 65 percent homology in *env* (K. Shimotohno, personal communication). This conservation of pX sequences supports the postulate that the pX region serves an important function for the virus.

As noted previously, three infectious clones of HTLV-II have been identified. λH-6 is the replication-competent wild-type virus, λH-9 and λH-2 are mutants which are probably replication incompetent, due to the deletion of critical structural gene information required for replication (Figure 1). These two mutants, however, conserved the bulk of the pX region. Of interest is the observation that the deletion mutants are present in the late passage, but not the early passage, Mo cells. The early passage Mo, which contains only wild-type HTLV-II, has very stringent growth requirements, while late passage Mo, which contains all three HTLV-II proviral forms, can grow in serum-free medium and will clone spontaneously at limiting dilution and in methylcellulose. These differences suggest that the HTLV-II deletion mutants might be causally related to the growth characteristics of late passage Mo, consistent with the hypothesis that the pX region is involved in HTLV-induced leukemogenesis (30). Neither specific mRNA transcripts nor protein products of the pX region have been identified for either HTLV-II or HTLV-I. Intensive investigative efforts are underway in several laboratories to define the significance of the pX region to the process of leukemic transformation and to identify, isolate, and characterize the putative pX gene products.

6. SUMMARY

HTLV-II is one of the two major types of a lymphotropic retrovirus that is epidemiologically associated with human T-lymphocyte malignancy. Despite the fact that HTLV-II has been noted in a single patient with a T-cell variant of hairy-cell leukemia, it exhibits virtually identical biological properties *in vitro* to those noted for HTLV-I, which is generally associated with highly aggressive disease. Molecular cloning of HTLV-II has revealed significant sequence differences between HTLV-II and HTLV-I. However, general structural features including proviral size, gene arrangement, and the presence of the pX region at the 3' end, are conserved. Sequence analysis of the LTR from HTLV-II and HTLV-I shows little overall homology, but does reveal the conservation of short sequences important for proviral integration, reverse transcription, and transcriptional regulation. The mechanism of HTLV-II-induced leukemic transformation is unknown, but indirect evidence suggest that the pX gene region is important to the process.

ACKNOWLEDGEMENT

We thank E. Koers for help in the preparation of this manuscript. Work was supported by NCI grants CA 30388, CA 32737, CA 09297 and CA 16042; and by grants PF-2182 and JFRA-99 from the American Cancer Society. Dr. William Wachsman is a Bank of America-Giannini Foundation Fellow.

REFERENCES

1. Poiesz BJ, Ruscetti FW, Gazdar AF, Bunn PA, Minna JD, Gallo RC: Detection and isolation of type C retrovirus particles from fresh and cultured lymphocytes of a patient with cutaneous T-cell lymphoma. Proc. Natl. Acad. Sci. USA 77: 7415-7419, 1980.
2. Hinuma Y, Nagata K, Hanaoka M, Nakai M, Matsumoto T, Kinoshita K-I, Shirakawa S, Miyoshi I: Adult T-cell leukemia: Antigen in an ATL cell line and detection of antibodies to the antigen in human sera. Proc. Natl. Acad. Sci. USA 78:6476-6480, 1981.
3. Blattner WA, Kalyanaraman VS, Robert-Guroff M, Lister TA, Galton DAG, Sarin PS, Crawford MH, Catovsky D, Greaves M, Gallo RC: The human type-C retrovirus, HTLV, in Blacks from the Caribbean region, and relationship to adult T-cell leukemia/lymphoma. Int. J. Cancer 30:257-264, 1982.
4. Saxon A, Stevens RH, Golde DW: T-lymphocyte variant of hairy-cell leukemia. Ann. Intern. Med. 88:323-326, 1978.
5. Saxon A, Stevens RH, Quan SG, Golde DW: Immunologic characterization of hairy cell leukemias in continuous culture. J. Immunol. 120:777-782, 1978.
6. Groopman JE, Lusis AJ, Weisbart RH, Griffin FM Jr, Golde DW: Human lymphokines: Insights gained from characterization of products from a T-lymphocyte cell line. Leukemia Rev. Internatl. 2:125-150, 1984.
7. Remold HG, Mednis A, Kawaguchi T, Bersch N, Golde DW: Production of migration-inhibitory factor by a human T-lymphoblast cell line. Cell Immunol. 78:305-313, 1983.
8. Golde DW, Bersch N, Quan SG, Lusis AJ: Production of erythroid-potentiating activity by a human T-lymphoblast cell line. Proc. Natl. Acad. Sci. USA 77:593-596, 1980.

9. Kalyanaraman VS, Sarngadharan MG, Robert-Guroff M, Miyoshi I, Blayney D, Golde D, Gallo RC: A new subtype of human T-cell leukemia virus (HTLV-II) associated with a T-cell variant of hairy cell leukemia. Science 218:571-573, 1982.
10. Uchiyama T, Yodoi J, Sagawa K, Takatsuki K, Uchino H: Adult T-cell leukemia: Clinical and hematologic features of 16 cases. Blood 50:481-492, 1977.
11. Shimoyama M, Minato K, Saito H, Kitahara T, Konda C, Nakazawa M, Ishihara K, Watanabe S, Inada N, Nagatani T, Deura K, Mikata A: Comparison of clinical, morphologic and immunologic characteristics of adult T-cell leukemia-lymphoma and cutaneous T-cell lymphoma. Jpn. J. Clin. Oncol. 9 (Suppl):357-372, 1979.
12. Bunn PA Jr, Schechter GP, Jaffe E, Blayney D, Young RC, Matthews MJ, Blattner W, Broder S, Robert-Guroff M, Gallo RC: Clinical course of retrovirus-associated adult T-cell lymphoma in the United States. N. Engl. J. Med. 309:257-264, 1983.
13. Wachsman W, Golde DW, Chen ISY: Hairy-cell leukemia and human T cell leukemia. Semin. Oncol. 11:446-450, 1984.
14. Chen ISY, McLaughlin J, Gasson JC, Clark SC, Golde DW: Molecular characterization of genome of a novel human T-cell leukemia virus. Nature 305:502-505, 1983.
15. Seiki M, Hattori S, Yoshida M: Human adult T-cell leukemia virus: Molecular cloning of the provirus DNA and the unique terminal structure. Proc. Natl. Acad. Sci. USA 79: 6899-6902, 1982.
16. Shimotohno K, Golde DW, Miwa M, Sugimura T, Chen ISY: Nucleotide sequence analysis of the long terminal repeat of human T-cell leukemia virus type II. Proc. Natl. Acad Sci. USA 81:1079-1083, 1984.
17. Miyoshi I, Kubonishi I, Yoshimoto S, Akagi T, Ohtsuki Y, Shiraishi Y, Nagata K, Hinuma Y: Type C virus particles in a cord T-cell line derived by co-cultivating normal human cord leukocytes and human leukemic T cells. Nature 294: 770-771, 1981.
18. Yamamoto N, Okada M, Koyanagi Y, Kannagi M, Hinuma Y: Transformation of human leukocytes by co-cultivation with an adult T cell leukemia virus producer cell line. Science 217:737-739, 1982.
19. Popovic M, Sarin PS, Robert-Guroff M, Kalyanaraman VS, Mann D, Minowada J, Gallo RC: Isolation and transmission of human retrovirus (human T-cell leukemia virus). Science 219:856-859, 1983.
20. Chen ISY, Quan SG, Golde DW: Human T-cell leukemia virus type II transforms normal human lymphocytes. Proc. Natl. Acad. Sci. USA 80:7006-7009, 1983.
21. Gasson JC, Chen ISY, Westbrook CA, Golde DW: Lymphokines and hematopoiesis. In: Normal and Neoplastic Hematopoiesis. UCLA Symposia on Molecular and Cellular Biology, New Series, Vol. 9. Golde DW, Marks PA, eds. Alan Liss, 1983, pp. 129-139.

22. Temin HM: Function of the retrovirus long terminal repeat. Cell 28:3-5, 1982.
23. Srinivasan A, Reddy EP, Dunn CY, Aaronson SA: Molecular dissection of transcriptional control elements within the long terminal repeat of the retrovirus. Science 223:286-289, 1984.
24. Chen ISY, McLaughlin J, Golde DW: Long terminal repeats of human T-cell leukemia virus II genome determine target cell specificity. Nature 309:276-279, 1984.
25. Khoury G, Gruss P: Enhancer elements. Cell 33:313-314, 1983.
26. Weiss R, Teich N, Varmus H, Coffin J, eds: RNA Tumor Viruses. Cold Spring Harbor Laboratory, 1982.
27. Hayward WS, Neel BG, Astrin SM: Activation of a cellular onc gene by promoter insertion in ALV-induced lymphoid leukosis. Nature 290:475, 1981.
28. Tsichlis PN, Strauss PG, Hu LF: A common region for proviral DNA integration in MoMuLV-induced rat thymic lymphomas. Nature 302:445-449, 1983.
29. Hahn B, Manzari V, Colombini S, Franchini G, Gallo RC, Wong-Staal F: Common site of integration of HTLV in cells of three patients with mature T-cell leukaemia-lymphoma: A retraction. Nature 305:340, 1983.
30. Seiki M, Hattori S, Hirayama Y, Yoshida M: Human adult T-cell leukemia virus: Complete nucleotide sequence of the provirus genome integrated in leukemia cell DNA. Proc. Natl. Sci. USA 80:3618-3622, 1983.

5

ONCOGENE EXPRESSION AND ARRANGEMENT IN HUMAN LEUKEMIA

Steven J. Collins, M.D.

1. INTRODUCTION

It is generally assumed that human cancer results from a genetic mutation or series of mutations. There is a great deal of indirect evidence supporting this hypothesis. Studies with the X-linked G-6-PD marker indicate that most human malignancies are clonal (1) suggesting the occurrence of a rare event(s) in their development. Individuals with inherited defects in DNA repair such as Bloom's syndrome and xeroderma pigmentosa are more susceptible to certain malignancies than normals (2). Most carcinogens or carcinogen metabolites are thought to act by binding to and altering DNA. Specific chromosome abnormalities are found in malignant cells but not in normal cells from patients with certain malignancies indicating the presence of specific genetic rearrangements in these particular cancers. However, until recently the specific genes effected by mutations producing cancer were completely unknown. This situation has changed remarkably in the past several years with the isolation and characterization of specific human genes (oncogenes) that may be intimately related to malignant transformation. Amplification, point mutations and chromosome rearrangements involving certain of these oncogenes have been described in various human malignancies including the leukemias.

2. ISOLATION OF HUMAN ONCOGENES

Human oncogenes have been isolated by two general techniques: 1) Molecular cloning of human genes homologous to the transforming genes of animal acute transforming RNA tumor viruses; and 2) molecular cloning of human tumor cell genes that are responsible for the *in vitro* transformation of mouse NIH3T3 cells.

The acute transforming RNA tumor viruses (retroviruses) have been isolated from various species including chickens, rodents, cats and monkeys (3). They are capable of transforming cultured animal cells *in vitro* and rapidly producing tumors when injected into the appropriate host animal. The specific DNA sequences that are responsible for the transforming capacity of these viruses have been identified and molecularly cloned. Similar sequences homologous to these viral transforming sequences are found in the DNA of normal uninfected host cells. It appears that these RNA tumor viruses have picked up specific host sequences ("proto-oncogenes"), the acquisition of which enables them to transform other cells (4). Moreover these specific oncogene sequences display striking species to species evolutionary conservation. For example, sequences homologous to *myc*, the oncogene of the MC-29 acute transforming retrovirus of chickens, are found in virtually all vertebrate species including man. Although the physiological role of the products of these oncogene sequences is largely unknown, the evolutionary conservation of these sequences suggests that they are playing some basic, important function perhaps related to control of cell proliferation and/or differentiation. By using the animal retrovirus transforming sequences as molecular probes, some 15 distinct human oncogenes have been molecularly cloned and characterized and their chromosomal position determined.

The other major approach to identifying human oncogenes has been through the technique of DNA-mediated transformation of cultured mouse NIH3T3 cells. These cells continuously proliferate in culture but form few spontaneous colonies in soft agar and are not tumorigenic in immunosuppressed mice. Upon incubation of these cells with DNA derived from certain human tumors under conditions which encourage mouse cell uptake of the human tumor DNA, a small percentage of the mouse cells develop a malignant phenotype: i.e., they readily form colonies in soft agar and become tumorigenic in immunosuppressed mice (5,6). The existence of human DNA in these transformed NIH3T3 mouse cells is readily demonstrated, and the human genes responsible for this transformation have been molecularly cloned. Some of these transforming genes have been identified as members of the _ras_ family of retroviral oncogenes that are homologous to the transforming sequences of the Kirsten and Harvey rat sarcoma viruses (8-11). However, as with other retroviral related oncogenes, _ras_ oncogenes are found in the DNA of normal non-malignant human cells, and such normal cell DNA does not transform NIH3T3 cells. Thus, there must be a difference in the _ras_ gene structure of normal human cells versus the malignant human cells whose _ras_ gene is capable of transforming mouse NIH3T3 cells. At least one such difference has been characterized and involves a single nucleotide base changed at amino acid 12 of the _ras_ gene product (12-14). The _ras_ gene in normal untransformed cells exhibits at this site the codon GGC coding for glycine while the activated _ras_ gene in certain tumors contains at this site the codon GTC coding for valine. Thus this single point mutation within the _ras_ gene in some presently unknown way dramatically alters the _ras_ gene product such that it becomes capable of transforming NIH3T3 cells.

The significance of the mouse NIH3T3 transformation assay and of the human oncogenes isolated through its use is somewhat unclear. Only DNA from malignant cells and cell lines has been shown to have transforming activity in the NIH3T3 assay. DNA from normal, non-malignant cells does not transform. However, only about 15 - 20% of human tumors tested demonstrate transforming activity (5). The NIH3T3 cells themselves are unusual in that they demonstrate indefinite cell replication _in vitro_.

In contrast, normal mouse fibroblasts, with a finite *in vitro* life span, are not transformed by individual oncogenes. It has been suggested that NIH3T3 cells have already undergone at least one genetic change leading to tumorigenesis. The addition of an activated oncogene may then provide a second genetic change resulting in overt malignancy (7).

3. NORMAL ROLE OF HUMAN ONCOGENES

The oncogenes isolated to date demonstrate a striking evolutionary conservation in genomic DNA from species to species suggesting that they play an important, fundamental biologic role in normal as well as malignant cells. Indeed active transcription of certain oncogenes has been demonstrated in various normal, non-malignant embryonic and adult tissues (15). One of the most important and exciting areas of present oncogene research involves defining the normal physiologic function of the oncogene products and determining how an alteration of such products might lead to tumor formation.

A number of the cellular oncogenes including *fes*, *src* and *abl* have been demonstrated to have the ability to phosphorylate proteins, particularly tyrosine residues, *in vitro* (3). The products of these particular oncogenes reside in the cytoplasm or cell membrane, but the identity of the physiological target or targets of these products is presently unclear. Another family of oncogenes exemplified by the *myc* oncogene have been demonstrated to have a nuclear location and may bind to DNA (16). The *myc* gene appears to be activated when normal cells are encouraged to divide (17) but its role in such cells is presently unknown. A relationship between certain oncogenes and certain physiologic growth factors has been demonstrated by the dramatic discovery that the predicted amino acid sequence of the *sis* oncogene product and the amino acid sequence of platelet-derived growth factor are virtually identical (18,19). More recently a similarity between the predicted amino acid sequence of the *erb-B* oncogene product and the amino acid sequence of a portion of the receptor for epidermal growth factor has been demonstrated (20). These discoveries strengthen the hypotheses that oncogenes in general code for important proteins involved in normal physiological functions. Alterations of such products may lead to malignant transformation. Such an alteration in tumor cells might involve enhanced expression of a particular oncogene product (a "quantitative" defect), expression of an altered oncogene product (a "qualitative" defect), expression of an oncogene product at an inappropriate time in the cell cycle (a "regulatory" defect) or a combination of the above.

4. AMPLIFICATION OF ONCOGENES IN HUMAN LEUKEMIC CELLS

The HL-60 cell line is a culture of malignant promyelocytes derived from the peripheral blood leukocytes of a patient with acute promyelocytic leukemia (21). These cells can be induced *in vitro* to terminally differentiate to mature granulocytes by a number of different compounds (22). Sequences related to the *c-myc* oncogene are amplified some 10-20 fold in the genomic DNA of the HL-60 cell line (23) (Fig. 1). This oncogene amplification is not an artifact of tissue culture since a similar degree of *myc* amplification was noted in the DNA of non-cultured leukemic cells of the patient from whom the HL-60 culture was derived (24). A quantitatively similar increase in *myc* related messenger RNA has also been noted in HL-60 cells (25), when compared with other leukemic cells as well as normal cells, indicating that increased expression of the *myc* oncogene accompanies the *myc* gene amplification of these cells.

K-562 is a Philadelphia chromosome-positive cell line derived from a patient with chronic myelogenous leukemia (CML) in blast crisis (26). Human cellular oncogene sequences (*c-abl*) homologous to transforming sequences of the mouse Abelson leukemia virus (*v-abl*) are amplified some 4-8 fold in this cell line (27) (Fig. 2). A similar increase in *c-abl* related messenger RNA is found in K-562. Unlike HL-60 the *myc* oncogene is not amplified in K-562.

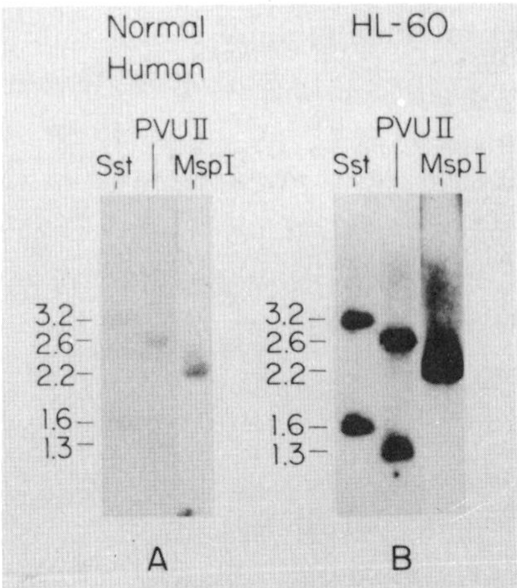

Figure 1: DNA from normal human peripheral blood cells and from HL-60 promyelocytic leukemia cells were digested with the indicated enzymes, subjected to agarose gel electrophoresis, blotted to nitrocellulose, and hybridized to a <u>myc</u> probe. The more intense signal of this probe hybridized to HL-60 DNA indicates amplification of <u>myc</u> related sequences in these leukemic cells.

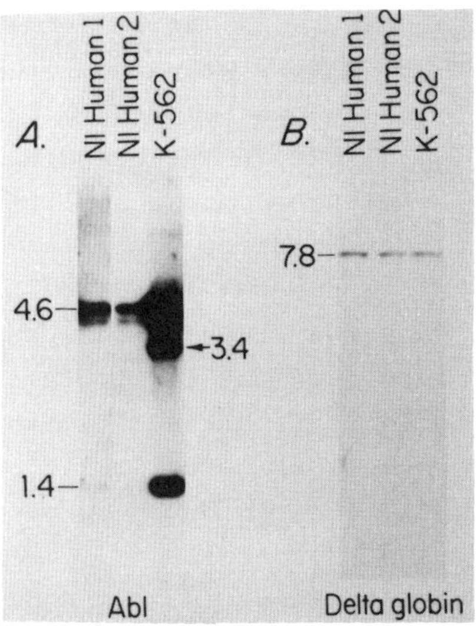

Figure 2: The indicated radiolabelled probes were sequentially hybridized to the same Southern transfer of Bgl II digests of K-562 and normal human DNA. The more intense hydridization of the <u>abl</u> probe to K-562 DNA indicates amplification of the <u>abl</u> sequences in this cell line.

The significance of oncogene amplification in these leukemic cell lines is unclear. Current speculation to explain malignant transformation includes the hypothesis that cancer results from an "overdose" of the products of cellular oncogenes (4). The amplification and increased expression of the <u>myc</u> and <u>abl</u> oncogenes in these cell lines is certainly consistent with this hypothesis. Interestingly, when HL-60 cells are induced to terminally differentiate to mature granulocytes, the level of myc messenger RNA markedly decreases in these cells (25). However, uncertainty with respect to the structure, function and physiological significance of the c-myc and c-abl protein products presently makes the "overdose" hypothesis difficult to confirm.

The amplification of oncogenes in leukemic cells appears to be an unusual event. We have not noted similar myc gene amplification in at least 20 other leukemic cells examined to date including some other promyelocytic leukemias. Similarly, we have not noted any other leukemic cells demonstrating c-abl gene amplification including several other CML blast crisis cell lines.

5. TRANSLOCATION OF ONCOGENES IN HUMAN LEUKEMIA

Both the myc and abl oncogenes are involved in specific chromosome translocations that characterize certain human lymphomas and leukemias. Over one half of the cases of Burkitt lymphoma exhibit a translocation between the q arms of chromosome 8 and 14. In many of these cases the c-myc oncogene which is normally located on the distal end of chromosome 8 is translocated into the immunoglobulin heavy chain locus located near the end of chromosome 14 (28,29). The chromosome breakpoints involved in such translocations are variable. In some cases the break on chromosome 8 occurs within the myc gene itself while in other cases the break occurs either 5' or 3' to the gene.

The significance of the myc gene translocation and how it relates to the pathogenesis of Burkitt lymphoma is presently unclear. In some Burkitt cell lines there is a marked increase in transcription of the translocated myc gene suggesting that the translocated gene has come under the influence of transcription enhancer elements normally present within the immunoglobulin heavy chain locus (30,31). In other Burkitt cell lines there is no marked increase in myc gene transcription but the translocated oncogene appears to have undergone numerous point mutations within its coding exons perhaps resulting in an altered myc gene product (32). Thus there is presently evidence both for a quantitative and qualitative change in the myc gene product as a result of the chromosomal translocation of this oncogene.

Over 90% of cases of CML exhibit the Philadelphia (Ph^1) chromosome which results from a reciprocal translocation between chromosomes 9 and 22. Recent studies have demonstrated that the c-abl oncogene, normally located on the distal end of chromosome 9, is translocated to the Philadelphia chromosome in cases of CML (33). In some cases of CML the break point on chromosome 9 is quite close to the c-abl oncogene (34). Interestingly, the translocation of c-abl occurs into a region of the q arm of chromosome 22 that may normally harbor the lambda light chain immunoglobulin locus, and both c-abl and lambda light chain genes are amplified to a similar degree in K-562 (27). However unlike the case of the myc oncogene in Burkitt lymphoma, there is presently no direct evidence that c-abl in CML is rearranged with any immunoglobulin sequences (35).

What are the consequences of the c-abl oncogene translocation in cases of CML? As with the myc translocation in Burkitt lymphoma this is a difficult question in light of present uncertainty with respect to the biological activity of the c-abl product. At the messenger RNA level we have found a predominant and novel 8.2 kb c-abl related RNA in four of four samples of Ph^1 positive CML cells and cell lines (Fig. 3). In addition the levels of abl related message are up to 8-fold higher in the CML blast crisis cells as compared with chronic phase CML and non-CML cells. Although there is presently no direct proof, it is possible that the translocation of c-abl in CML results in altered transcription of the c-abl locus manifest by the appearance of the novel 8.2 kb message. Such an altered transcript might give rise to an abnormal c-abl product that could somehow relate to the pathogenesis of CML.

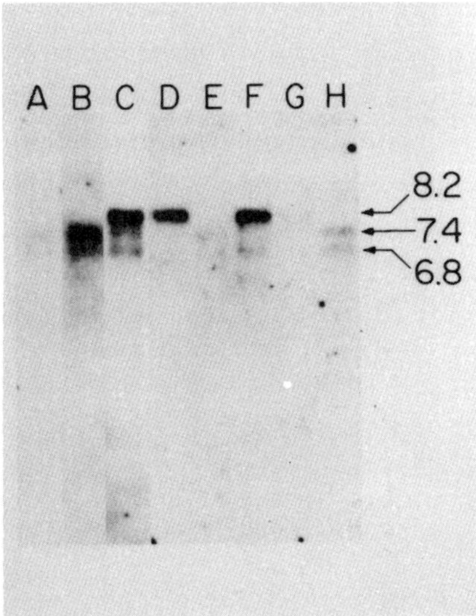

Figure 3: Poly A^+ RNA was isolated from the indicated cells, electrophoresed through 1% agarose, 2.2M formaldehyde gels, and blotted to a nitrocellulose filter. The filter was then hybridized to a radiolabelled abl probe. Cells are as follows: (A) HL-60 promyelocytic leukemia; (B) EBV transformed lymphocytes; (C) K-562; (D) EM-2, a CML blast crisis cell line; (E) Raji (Burkitt lymphoma); (F) KCL-22, a CML blast crisis cell line; (G) peripheral blood cells from a patient with Ph^1 positive CML; (H) KG-1, a myelogenous leukemia cell line.

6. MULTIPLE ONCOGENE ACTIVATION IN INDIVIDUAL LEUKEMIAS

Evidence is accumulating that more than one oncogene may be altered or activated in an individual leukemia. For example DNA from the HL-60 promyelocytic leukemia cell line which exhibits amplification of the c-myc oncogene (see above) is capable of transforming mouse NIH3T3 cells (6). However, the gene responsible for this transformation has been isolated and is clearly not c-myc but rather is a member of the ras oncogene family (N-ras) (36). Thus two genetic events involving oncogenes have been documented in HL-60: 1) amplification of c-myc, and 2) activation of the N-ras gene perhaps by a point mutation. Similarly, certain Burkitt lymphoma cell lines which display an 8:14 translocation can transform NIH3T3 cells but the activated gene responsible for this transformation (B-lym) is clearly distinct from the translocated c-myc gene (37). These results indicate that more than one oncogene may be altered or activated in an individual tumor. Moreover, some in vitro experiments also suggest that malignant transformation requires the activation of at least two types of oncogenes. Rat embryo fibroblasts, which unlike NIH3T3 cells have a finite life span in culture (and thus more closely resemble normal, untransformed cells), cannot be malignantly transformed by individual oncogenes. However, such cells can be transformed by a combination of transfected oncogenes such as _myc_ and _ras_ (38). These experiments are consistent with the hypothesis that there are multiple stages in the pathogenesis of malignancy and that cancer results not from a single mutation but from a series of successive mutations.

REFERENCES

1. Fialkow PJ: Clonal origin of human tumors. Biochem. Biophys. Acta. 458:283-321, 1976.
2. Knudson AG: Genetic factors in human malignancy. Advances in Human Genetics, Harris H (ed), pp. 1-51, 1977.
3. Bishop JM: Oncogenes. Scientific American 246:80-94, 1982.
4. Bishop JM: Enemies within: The genesis of retrovirus oncogenes. Cell 23:5-6, 1981.
5. Cooper GM: Cellular transforming genes. Science 217:801-806, 1982.
6. Murray MJ, Shilo B-Z, Shih C, Cowing D, Hsu HW, Weinberg RA: Three different human tumor cell lines contain different oncogenes. Cell 25:355-361, 1981.
7. Weinberg RA: A molecular basis of cancer. Scientific American 249:126-142, 1983.
8. Der C, Krontiris T, Cooper G: Transforming genes of human bladder and lung carcinoma lines are homologous to the _ras_ genes of Harvey and Kirsten sarcoma viruses. Proc. Natl. Acad. Sci. USA 79:3637-3640, 1982.
9. Parada L, Tabin C, Shih C, Weinberg R: Human EJ bladder carcinoma oncogene is homologue of Harvey sarcoma virus _ras_ gene. Nature 297:474-478, 1982.
10. Santos E, Tronick S, Aaronson S, Pulciani S, Barbacid M: The T24 human bladder carcinoma oncogene is an activated form of the normal human homologue of Balb and Harvey-MSV transforming genes. Nature 298:343-347, 1982.
11. Shimizu et al: Three human transforming genes are related to the viral _ras_ oncogenes. Proc. Natl. Acad. Sci. USA 80:2112-2116, 1983.

12. Tabin C, Bradley D, Bargmann C, Weinberg R, Papageorge A, Scolnick E, Dhar R, Lowy D, Chang E: Mechanism of activation of a human oncogene. Nature 300:143-149, 1982.
13. Reddy E, Reynolds R, Santos E, Barbacid M: A point mutation is responsible for the acquisition of transforming properties by the T24 bladder carcinoma oncogene. Nature 300:149-155, 1982.
14. Taparowsky E, Suard Y, Fascuro O, Shimizu K, Goldfarb M, Wigler M: Activation of the T24 bladder carcinoma transforming gene is linked to a single amino acid change. Nature 300:762-765, 1982.
15. Muller R, Tremblay JM, Adamson ED, Verma I: Tissue and cell-type specific expression of two human c-onc genes. Nature 304:454-456, 1983.
16. Hann S, Abrams H, Rohrschneider L, Eisenman R: Proteins encoded by v-myc and c-myc oncogenes: Identification and localization in acute leukemia virus transformants and bursal lymphoma cell lines. Cell (in press).
17. Kelly K, Cochran B, Stiles C, Leder P: Cell-specific regulation of the c-myc gene by lymphocyte mitogens and platelet derived growth factor. Cell 35:603-610, 1983.
18. Waterfield MD, Scrace GT, Whittle N, Stroobant P, Johnsson, A, Wasteson A, Westermark B, Heldin C, Huang J, Devel T: Platelet-derived growth factor is structurally related to the putative transforming protein $p28^{sis}$ of simian sarcoma virus. Nature 304:35-39, 1983.
19. Doolittle R, Hunkapillar M, Hood L, Devare S, Robbins K, Aaronson S, Antoniades H: Simian sarcoma virus onc gene, v-sis is derived from the gene (or genes) encoding a platelet-derived growth factor. Science 221:275-277, 1983.
20. Downward J, Yarden Y, Mayes E, Scrace G, Totty N, Stockwell P, Ullrich A, Schlessinger J, Waterfield M: Close similarity of epidermal growth factor receptor and v-erb B oncogene protein sequences. Nature 307:521-527, 1984.
21. Collins S, Gallo R, Gallagher R: Continuous growth and differentiation of human myeloid leukemia cells in suspension culture. Nature 270:347-349, 1977.
22. Collins S, Ruscetti F, Gallagher R, Gallo R: Terminal differentiation of human promyelocytic leukemia induced by dimethylsulfoxide and other polar compounds. Proc. Natl. Acad. Sci. USA 75:2458-2462, 1978.
23. Collins S, Groudine M: Amplification of endogenous myc-related sequences in a human myeloid leukemia cell line. Nature 298:679-681, 1982.
24. Dalla-Favera R, Wong-Staal F, Gallo R: Onc gene amplification of promyelocytic leukemia cell line HL-60 and primary leukemia cells of the same patient. Nature 299: 61-63, 1982.
25. Westin E et al: Expression of cellular homologues of retroviral onc genes in human hematopoietic cells. Proc. Natl. Acad. Sci. USA 79:2490-2494, 1982.

26. Lozzio CB, Lozzio BB: Human chronic myelogenous leukemia cell line with positive Philadelphia chromosome. Blood 45:321-334, 1975.
27. Collins S, Groudine M: Rearrangement and amplification of c-abl sequences in the human chronic myelogenous leukemia cell line K-562. Proc. Natl. Acad. Sci. USA 80:4813-4817, 1983.
28. Dalla-Favera R et al: Human c-myc oncogene is located on the region of chromosome 8 that is translocated in Burkitt lymphoma cells. Proc. Natl. Acad. Sci. USA 79:7824-7827, 1982.
29. Taub R et al: Translocation of the c-myc gene into the immunoglobulin heavy chain locus in human Burkitt lymphoma and mouse plasmacytoma cells. Proc. Natl. Acad. Sci. USA 79:7837-7841, 1982.
30. Erikson J, AR-Rushdi A, Drwinga H, Nowell P, Croce C: Transcriptional activation of the translocated c-myc oncogene in Burkitt lymphoma. Proc. Natl. Acad. Sci. USA 80: 820-824, 1983.
31. Hayday A, Gillies S, Saito H, Wood C, Wiman K, Hayward W, Tonegawa S: Activation of a translocated c-myc gene by an enhancer in the immunoglobulin heavy chain locus. Nature 307:334-340, 1984.
32. Rabbitts T, Hamlyn P, Baer R: Altered nucleotide sequences of a translocated c-myc gene in Burkitt lymphoma. Nature 306:760-765, 1983.
33. deKlein A et al: A cellular oncogene is translocated to the Philadelphia chromosome in chronic myelocytic leukemia. Nature 300:765-767, 1982.
34. Heisterkamp N, Stephenson J, Groffen J, Hansen P, deKlein A, Bartram C, Grosveld G: Localization of the c-abl oncogene adjacent to a translocation breakpoint in chronic myelocytic leukemia. Nature 306:239-242, 1983.
35. Groffen J, Stephenson J, Heisterkamp N, deKlein A, Bartram C, Grosveld G: Philadelphia chromosome breakpoints are clustered within a limited region, bcr, on chromosome 22. Cell 36:93-99, 1984.
36. Murray M, Cunningham J, Parada L, Dantry F, Lebowitz P, Weinberg R: The HL-60 transforming sequence: A ras oncogene coexisting with altered myc gene in hematopoietic tumors. Cell 33:749-757, 1983.
37. Diamond A, Cooper G, Ritz J, Lane M: Identification and molecular cloning of the human Blym transforming gene activated in Burkitt's lymphomas. Nature 305:112-116, 1983.
38. Land H, Parada L, Weinberg R: Tumorigenic conversion of primary embryo fibroblasts requires at least two cooperating oncogenes. Nature 304:596-602, 1983.

6

CLONAL VARIATION AND PHENOTYPIC PROGRESSION IN RETROVIRUS TRANSFORMED LEUKEMIA CELLS

Dr. David L. Hines

Relationships between *in vitro* growth factor autonomy, replicative capacity, differentiation, and leukemogenicity were investigated using murine myelogenous leukemia cells derived from Abelson virus (A-MuLV) leukemic mice and interleukin-3 dependent hemopoietic cells infected *in vitro* with A-MuLV. All promonocytic cell lines cloned from A-MuLV leukemic mice were growth factor independent *in vitro*, and tumorigeneic *in vivo*. Separate, cloned lines from individual leukemic mice differed in their responsiveness to granulocyte-macrophage colony stimulating activity (GM-CSA), and in their capacity to differentiate. Differentiation of cloned lines *in vitro* led to a reduction of *in vitro* replicative capacity and tumorigenicity. However, clonal lines which did not differentiate *in vitro*, in response to GM-CSA, were isolated from all leukemias. Growth factor dependent, non-leukemogenic hemopoietic progenitor cells (FDPC), derived from long term bone marrow cultures, were grown in interleukin-3 containing conditioned medium and infected with A-MuLV. Growth-factor independent colony forming cells could be identified as early as one week after infection. The growth factor autonomous cells produced A-MuLV, GM-CSA, a beta-type transforming growth factor activity, and were able to support the growth of factor dependent FDPC. However, the loss of *in vitro* growth-factor dependency in these autonomous lines was not analogous to acquisition of *in vivo* tumorigenicity, for less than 10% of syngeneic mice inoculated with growth-factor autonomous cells developed progressively growing tumors.

1. INTRODUCTION

Clinical observations have indicated neoplasms can undergo changes over time which usually result in an increase in growth and metastatic potentials. This phenomenon, termed neoplastic progression, has been defined as acquisition of permanent, irreversible, qualitative changes in one or more characteristics in a neoplasm (1). The loss or acquisition of individual characteristics can occur independently over protracted periods of time. While there is considerable evidence that most human leukemias are clonal neoplasms, i.e., they originate from transformation of a single cell (2), analysis of individual leukemic cells at the time of clinical diagnosis often indicates considerable heterogeneity (3,4), and additional neoplastic progression frequently occurs after the diagnosis, particularly in chronic myelogenous leukemia (5). Although the molecular lesions responsible for leukemic transformation are still not well understood, examination of leukemic cells and cell lines derived from the overt leukemic period have indicated several characteristics commonly found in leukemia: (1) the acquisition of increased proliferative potential, (2) a relative unresponsiveness to normal control limits so that the leukemic population density exceeds that of normal cells; and (3) a reduced ability to undergo normal maturation. Examination of overtly leukemic cells is, however, unlikely to be informative about the events preceeding full expression of malignancy.

Investigations of the cellular mechanisms involved in expression of leukemogenicity would benefit from the availability of an *in vitro* method for reproduction of the transforming event(s) which culminates in the production of overtly leukemic cells similar to those induced *in vivo* by the same leukemogen. The murine long term bone marrow culture system (LTBMC) as originally described by Dexter et al. (6,7) and modified by Greenberger (8), allows the production of hemopoietic stem cells for months, and is a particularly attractive focus for developing an *in vitro* model of myeloid leukemogenesis. In the LTBMC stem cell differentiation occurs primarily along the granulocyte-macrophage lineage (7). Additionally, culture of cells removed from LTBMC with interleukin-3 can produce long-term, growth-factor dependent hemopoietic cell lines referred to as FDPC (9-12). These non-malignant FDPC lines may be committed to a single pathway of differentiation, usually myeloid or basophil/mast cell, or show evidence of multipotential differentiation to erythroid, myeloid, and mast cell types (9-12). Abelson murine leukemia virus (A-MuLV), a replication defective retrovirus with a defined oncogene (v-abl) and oncogene product (13,14), can transform hemopoietic cells both *in vivo* and *in vitro* (15). The cell type most commonly described as transformed by A-MuLV *in vivo* resembles a pre-B lymphocyte (16), however we have recently described the frequent isolation of promonocytic leukemia cells from A-MuLV leukemic mice (17), confirming the ability of A-MuLV to transform monocytic linage cells (18). In an effort to study events preceeding the appearance of overtly leukemic cells, we have been investigating growth-factor autonomy, changes in capacity for differentiation, and leukemogenicity of FDPC cells infected *in vitro* by A-MuLV. The properties of these cells have been compared to those of promonocytic leukemic cells derived from A-MuLV leukemic mice. The results indicate that the acquisition of *in vitro* growth factor autonomy is not alone sufficient for expression of *in vivo* leukemogenicity.

2. MATERIALS AND METHODS

2.1 Mice and viruses

Inbred BALB/c mice, specific pathogen free, were maintained at the Michigan Cancer Foundation by brother-sister mating of stock originally obtained from Charles River Breeding Laboratories. The Abelson virus stocks used were prepared by infection of ANN-1 transformed non-producer cells with the helper virus (RF-MuLV) isolated from the regressing strain of Friend virus, and were assayed as has been described (17).

2.2 Long term bone marrow cultures

LTBMC were established in a manner similar to that described by Dexter (6) and modified by Greenberger (8). Briefly, bone marrow cells were flushed from femurs of BALB/c mice using RPMI 1640 medium supplemented with 15% horse serum, 10% fetal calf serum, 10^{-7} M hydrocortisone sodium succinate, 50 uM 2-mercaptoethanol, and 5 ug/ml gentamycin. 10^7 cells were cultured in 5 ml of the above medium in 25 cm^2 culture flasks at 33°C in 5% CO_2 in air. For the first 3 weeks the cultures were fed and depopulated at weekly intervals by replacing 2.5 ml of medium. After 3 weeks all of the medium was replaced at weekly intervals. With this system recharging with fresh bone marrow cells is not necessary and hemopoiesis has been maintained in some cultures for over 12 months.

FDPC cell lines were established from the nonadherent cells present in the medium removed during feeding. The cells were centrifuged (500 g, 5 min) and resuspended in the growth medium described above. Aliquots of cells were plated at $2x10^5$ cells/ml in 5ml of growth medium alone, growth medium supplemented with 10% conditioned medium from pokeweed mitogen stimulated spleen cells (PWMSCM), growth medium supplemented with 10% conditioned medium (CM) from the WEHI-3 murine myelomonocytic leukemia cell line (WEHI-3CM), or growth medium supplemented with 10% CM from the 266AD murine bone marrow preadipocyte cell line (19). The preparation of PWMSCM and 266AD CM have been described (19) and WEHI-3 CM was prepared as described by Dexter et al. (9). The cells were cultured at 37°C in an atmosphere of 5% CO_2 in air. Cultures were subcultured at least weekly by transfer of nonadherent or loosely adherent cells into fresh medium, maintaining cell concentrations below $5x10^5$ cells/ml.

2.3 Infection of FDPC and LTBMC cells

FDPC cells and nonadherent cells from LTBMC were centrifuged (500 g, 5 min) and 10^6 cells resuspended in 0.5 ml of growth medium containing 4 ug/ml polybrene. The resuspended cells were then mixed with 0.5 ml of at least 10^6 focus forming units of RF (A-MuLV) contained in Dulbecco's modified Eagles medium (DMEM) supplemented with 10% calf serum. Control cells were mixed with DMEM plus 10% calf serum alone. The 1.0 ml virus and cell mixtures were incubated at 37°C in a water bath for 2 hours, then diluted with 4.0 ml growth medium containing either 10% PWMSCM or 10% WEHI-3 CM, transferred to 25 cm^2 tissue culture flasks, and incubated at 37°C in an atmosphere of 5% CO_2 in air.

2.4 Agar culture methods

The method used for assaying granulocyte-macrophage colony stimulating activity (GM-CSA) by culture of normal bone marrow cells in semisolid agar cultures has been described (19). The culture of A-MuLV transformed leukemia lines in agar, and the method of scoring colonies for content of differentiated cells based on colony morphology was done as previously described from this laboratory (19).

2.5 Soft agar assay for transforming growth factors

Clone 49F, normal rat kidney fibroblasts (ATCC CRL 1570) was used for assaying transforming growth factors in a modification of the procedure described by DeLarco and Todaro (23). Briefly, 10^3 49F cells/ml were suspended in the samples to be tested in 0.3% agar (Difco) in DMEM (GIBCO) supplemented with 10% calf serum (GIBCO) and 5 ug/ml gentamycin. Aliquots (1.0 ml) of this mixture were pipetted onto a 1.0 ml base layer of 0.5% agar in DMEM with 10% calf serum in 35 mm petri dishes. Plates were incubated 10 days at 37°C in a humidified 5% CO_2 atmosphere in air. The assay was read unfixed and unstained, using a dissecting microscope with a calibrated ocular micrometer, counting all colonies larger than 0.10 mm. Where indicated epidermal growth factor (EGF) (Sigma) at 2 ng/ml was included in the test media. EGF alone at 2 ng/ml produced an average of only four colonies per thousand greater than 0.10 mm and only $10/10^3$ between 0.05 and 0.10 mm.

3. RESULTS

3.1 Characteristics of A-MuLV transformed promonocytic leukemia cells from leukemic animals

The origin and method of establishment of monocytic linage cell lines from RF (A-MuLV) leukemic BALB/c mice has been reported (17). During the initial 2 to 3 months at each subculturing a declining rate of spontaneous differentiation to apparent mature, adherent, phagocytic macrophages was noticed. Eventually the cell lines resembled very immature monoblasts or promonocytes which were weakly phagocytic, non-specific esterase positive, produced small amounts of lysozyme, expressed low levels of Fc and complement receptors, and were H-2 antigen positive but Ia antigen negative. All lines were initiated and grew in RPMI 1640 medium supplemented with 10% fetal calf serum, 10% calf serum, and 50 uM 2-mercaptoethanol only, with no additional requirements for external sources of hemopoietic growth factors. All lines were highly tumorigenic in syngeneic mice, inducing death within 3 weeks following subcutaneous inoculation of $5x10^5$ cells.

The very heterogeneous primary cultures could be maintained for a prolonged period by continued replacement of part of the medium. When cells from the primary cultures were cultured in 0.3% agar, both with and without 10% PWMSCM or 10% 266AD CM, colonies composed of both immature blast-like cells and more differentiated macrophages were observed. However, subculturing of agar colonies produced only lines composed of immature cells which resembled the lines produced by continued subculturing of primary cultures as described above. These observations were repeated with cells from individual leukemic mice, suggesting the more mature cells in the heterogeneous populations were capable of only limited growth, and that differentiation of the leukemic cells was accompanied by a reduction in replicative capacity.

Examination of 25 promonocytic lines, derived from colonies of cells from 5 separate leukemic mice, indicated that while all had many similar characteristics, they differed significantly in their ability to differentiate when cultured with various sources of granulocyte-macrophage colony stimulating factors (GM-CSF) (19 and D.L. Hines, unpublished observations). These lines were derived from individual agar colonies and were presumed to be clonal in origin. When these clonal lines were recultured in agar in the presence or absence of GM-CSF; (1) 17 lines produced an increased frequency of colonies containing differentiated cells in the presence of GM-CSF (2); 5 lines produced a low number of colonies containing differentiated cells whether or not GM-CSF was present; (3), and 3 lines never produced any differentiated cells. Clonal lines of all three of these types were isolated from 3 of 5 leukemic mice.

To investigate the relationship between differentiation and replicative capacity, three clonal lines from the same mouse, each representative of one of the three types described above, were cultured in 0.3% agar for seven days with and without 266AD CM as a source of GM-CSF. After seven days the colonies were counted and scored as containing differentiated or undifferentiated cells based on colony morphology as described (19). Individual colonies of each type were then removed from the agar and both the total cell number, and the number of cells capable of forming colonies when recultured in agar (2° CFU), were determined. As shown in Table 1, with both the AC5 and the AC8 cell line the average colony size and the content of 2° CFU per colony was significantly less ($p<0.05$) in differentiated colonies than in undifferentiated colonies. The AC5 cell line spontaneously produces differentiated colonies in agar, but is unresponsive to any source of GM-CSF we have tested. In contrast, the AC8 cell line produces an increased number of differentiated colonies when cultured with 266AD CM as a source of

GM-CSF (19). The C11 cell line has not been observed to produce differentiated cells when cultured with or without GM-CSF. We have interpreted the results showing a reduction in colony size and in the number of cells capable of secondary colony formation within agar colonies containing differentiated cells, as indicating maturation is accompanied by a reduced replicative capacity *in vitro*.

Table 1

Comparison of Colony Size and 2° CFU Content of Agar Culture Colonies of Clonal Cell Lines

Cell Line	Undifferentiated Colonies			Differentiated Colonies			Ratio Undiff./Diff.	
	Colony Size ($x10^{-3}$)	2°CFU/10^3 Cells	Total 2°CFU	Colony Size ($x10^{-3}$)	2°CFU/10^3 Cells	Total 2°CFU	Colony Size	Total 2°CFU
AC5								
Expt. 1 (5)[a]	48.0[b]	56±92[c]	2688	19.0	11±10	209	2.5	12.9
Expt. 2 (45)	11.7	384±116	4493	5.4	146±56	788	2.2	5.7
Expt. 3 (5)	13.0±5.0	271±26	3523	3.7±1.15	146±49	540	3.5	6.5
Expt. 4 (60)	12.5	599±95	7488	5.5	156±14	858	2.3	8.7
Expt. 5 (10)	18.5	681±41	12,803	7.6	299±51	2272	2.5	5.6
AC8								
Expt. 1 (6)	52.0±31	28±7	1457	35.0±27	8±7	280	1.5	5.2
Expt. 2 (5)	10.0±5.4	143±84	1430	8.1±8.4	149±129	1207	1.2	1.2
Expt. 3 (5)	16.5±4.7	352±255	5808	7.8±0.4	96±87	749	2.1	7.8
C11								
Expt. 1 (20)	17.4	209±41	3637	None observed				

[a] Number of colonies of each type used in this experiment.

[b] Average cell number; standard deviation given only when colonies were counted separately.

[c] Average ± standard deviation.

To determine if a reduced replicative capacity *in vitro* is reflected in a reduction in *in vivo* tumorgenicity, graded numbers of cells from differentiated and undifferentiated colonies were inoculated subcutaneously into syngeneic mice and the animals observed for tumor development. To simplify interpretation of the origin of late arising tumors, all *in vivo* studies were done with the AC5 cells which no longer produce infectious A-MuLV, but still produce non-infectious particles. As shown in

Figure 1, at low doses cells from differentiated colonies were less tumorigeneic than cells from undifferentiated colonies. This indicated a reduction in _in vitro_ replicative capacity was correlated with a reduction in tumorigenicity.

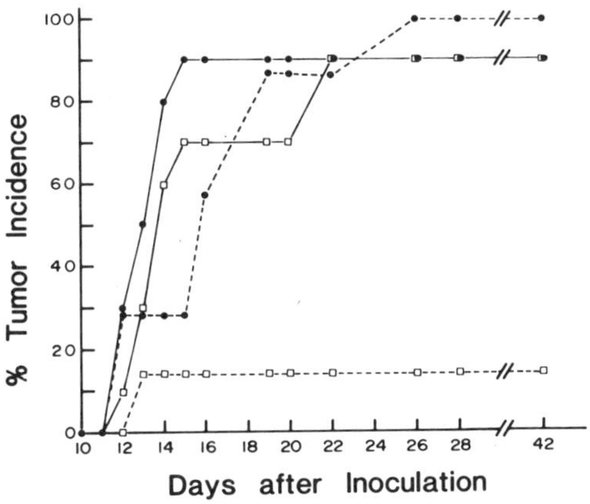

Figure 1. Occurence of tumors in syngeneic mice inoculated subcutaneously with A-MuLV induced AC5 cells from undifferentiated (——) or differentiated (----) agar colonies; (●) $2.1x10^3$ cells, (□) $7x10^2$ cells.

3.2 <u>In vitro A-MuLV infection of factor-dependent hemopoietic cells</u>

Growth of non-adherent cells removed from LTBMC at weekly demipopulations was dependent upon supplementation of the medium with additional growth factors. As indicated in Table 2 both PWMSCM and WEHI-3 CM were adequate sources of growth factors for these cells but 266AD CM was not. The growth factor (presumably interleukin-3) dependency of subcultured, non-adherent cells was absolute regardless if they were removed 1 week or 12 months after establishment of the LTBMC. Morphological examination of the factor-dependent cells during the first 3 or 4 subcultures indicated most were early cells of the myelomonocytic linage with a minor proportion (<10%) appearing to be basophils or mast cells, and the rest more mature neutrophils or monocytes. With continued subculturing up to 90% eventually resembled immature myelomonocytic linage cells which we have referred to as factor-dependent precursor cells, FDPC.

Table 2

Growth of LTBMC Nonadherent Cells Subcultured with Various Conditioned Media

Expt.	Medium Supplement	Cell count/ml x 10^{-5} at each weekly subculture[a]									
		1	2	3	4	5	6	7	8	9	10
1	None	0.04	<0.01	---							
	10% PWMSCM	6.7	3.4	5.5	3.9	4.0	4.9	1.8	3.1	1.9	3.5
	10% 266ADCM	1.6	1.5	0.4	<0.01	---					
2	None	0.1	<0.01	---							
	10% PWMSCM	4.7	1.6	1.2	2.8	3.1	1.9	2.3	2.5		
3	None	0.2	<0.01	---	---	---	---				
	10% WEHI-3CM	2.1	2.2	1.4	2.5	3.6	2.4				
	10% PWMSCM	2.4	2.5	1.3	1.2	3.4	1.8				

[a] Concentration adjusted to 2 x 10^5/ml initially and at each subculture.

FDPC derived from LTBMC between 1 and 4 weeks after initiation were infected with RF (A-MuLV) following 1 to 9 weeks of factor-dependent growth. After RF (A-MuLV) infection the cells continued to be cultured in the presence of 10% PWMSCM or WEHI-3 CM, otherwise the infected cells died within 2-4 days as did uninfected FDPC. At 1, 3, and 5 weeks after infection, cells were cultured in 0.3% agar in the absence of growth factor containing conditioned medium, and the number of 7 day growth factor independent colonies was determined (Table 3). Three weeks after infection, production of both infectious A-MuLV and the RF (MuLV) helper virus was determined. In the 4 experiments shown in Table 3, in which productive A-MuLV infection occurred, growth factor independent colonies were detected by week 3. In contrast, productive helper virus infection alone (#340B-1) did not support factor independent colony formation. In 3 of 4 experiments A-MuLV producing liquid cultures could be subpassaged without PWMSCM or WEHI-3 CM by week 5 after infection, and were therefore growth factor independent. Growth factor independency was not achieved by the 349B cells which eventually stopped producing infectious A-MuLV. Phenotypic characteristics of both uninfected and A-MuLV producing growth factor independent FDPC 8 weeks after infection are shown in Table 4. Infected 340-1 cells appear to express more differentiation markers than their uninfected 340A counterparts, while marker expression of the 421B1 and 421B2 cells was less consistent.

Table 3

Virus Production, Growth-Factor Independent Colony Formation, and Tumorigenicity of Uninfected and A-MuLV Infected FDPC

	Virus Production[a]			Number of Growth Factor Independent Agar Colonies per 10^5 Cells			
				Weeks After Infection			
Cells	Virus	Abelson Virus FFU/ml	Helper Virus PFU/ml	1	3	5	Tumorigenicity[b]
340A	None	0	0	N.D.	0	0	0/8
340A-1	A-MuLV	2.5×10^2	$>10^3$	N.D.	128	211	0/47
340B	None	0	0	0	0	0	0/10
340B-1	A-MuLV	0	300	0	0	0	0/10
349A	None	0	N.D.	0	40	0	N.D.
349B	A-MuLV	75	N.D.	2	80	28	N.D.
358A	None	C	N.D.	0	N.D.	0	0/6
358B	A-MuLV	8.5×10^6	N.D.	627	N.D.	1198	4/16
421B2	None	0	0	0	0	0	0/10
421B1	A-MuLV	5.5×10^2	$>10^3$	129	43	460	0/15

[a] Virus titers determined 3 weeks after infection, using NIH/3T3 cells for Abelson virus and XC cells for the helper virus.

[b] Number of animals developing subcutaneous tumors following inoculation with 1-5 x 10^6 cells over the total number of animals inoculated.

[c] Not tested.

Beginning 6 weeks after infection, 1-5x10^6 growth-factor independent cells and uninfected FDPC were inoculated subcutaneously into normal 8-10 week old syngeneic BALB/c mice, and the animals observed for up to 6 months for signs of local or systemic tumor growth or leukemia (Table 3). Tumor growth was seen in only 4 of 16 animals receiving 3x10^6 358B cells and 0 of 62 animals receiving between 1-5x10^6 340A-1 or 421B1 cells. The four tumors which did develop were small and only 2 of the 4 grew progressively. Thus, for these in vitro A-MuLV infected FDPC acquisition of growth factor autonomy in vitro was not sufficient for progressive growth in vivo.

Table 4

Characteristics of Uninfected and A-MuLV Infected FDPC

Characteristic	Uninfected FPDC		A-MuLV Infected FDPC		
	340A	421B2	340A-1	358B	421B1
% with Fc Receptor	1.5%	N.D.[a]	44.5%	N.D.	N.D.
% Phagocytic (latex beads)	1.4%	1.0%	68.5%	13.5%	4.0%
Lysozyme Secreted Per 10^5 cells	1.31 ug	19.0 ug	11.18 ug	1.8 ug	9.4 ug
Non-specific Esterase Positive	8%	43.5%	82%	95%	11.5%
Napthol AS-D Chloroacetate Esterase Positive	17%	27.4%	89%	12%	44.8%
% Histamine Positive	1.2%	5.7%	>0.1%	>0.1%	1.7%

[a] Not done.

3.3 Growth factor production by A-MuLV infected FDPC

The production of soluble growth regulators by A-MuLV infected FDPC was investigated because autostimulation of growth has been reported for both human (20) and murine myelogenous leukemia cell lines (21), and autocrine secretion of growth regulators has been suggested as a mechanism by which leukemic cells can obtain growth factor independency. No evidence of autostimulation of growth was seen when 340A-1 cells were cultured in 0.3% agar at increasing concentrations of cells, i.e., plating efficiency, as determined by the number of 7 day colonies, was independent of cell concentration between 25 and 5000 cells/ml. Furthermore, plating efficiency was not affected by culture of 340A-1 cells in agar in the presence of 340A-1 conditioned media at concentrations ranging from 0.5% to 40%. These experiments gave no indication of the type of autostimulation of growth which has been reported for both human HL-60 (20) and murine myelogenous leukemia cell lines (21).

Conditioned medium (CM) from 340A-1 cells was tested for its ability to support the growth of both normal bone marrow cells and uninfected growth factor dependent 340A cells (Table 5).

Table 5

Growth Supporting Activity of Conditioned Medium from Uninfected and A-MuLV Infected FDPC

	Agar Culture Colonies/10^5 Cells[a]	
Conditioned Medium[b]	Normal Bone Marrow Cells	FDPC (340A)
340A (FDPC)	31 ± 12	0 ± 0
340A-1 (A-MuLV infected FDPC)[c]	82 ± 9[d]	43 ± 8[d]
L-Cell	244 ± 49	N.D.[e]
Media Control[f]	22 ± 8	>1000
None	0 ± 0	0 ± 0

[a] Mean ± standard deviation

[b] Medium from cultures 3 days after initiation at 2 x 10^5/ml, tested at 10% v/v.

[c] 340A-1 tested 12 weeks after A-MuLV infection.

[d] Significantly different from 340A and media control by t Test, $p < 0.001$

[e] N.D. = Not done

[f] Media control for normal bone marrow, growth media with 1% PWMSCM; for FDPC, growth media with 10% PWMSCM.

Conditioned medium from 340A-1 cells, cultured for three days in RPMI 1640, was compared to medium from 340A cells cultured for 3 days in the presence of 10% PWMSCM. CM from 340A-1 cells cultured without PWMSCM supported the growth of approximately 1/3 as many bone marrow colonies as did L cell CM, a positive control. This was a significant increase over the number of colonies produced by 340A CM and the medium control. All colonies were composed of granulocytes, macrophages or both. These results indicated the production of soluble granulocyte-macrophage colony stimulating factor by the growth factor independent cells. Furthermore, CM from 340A-1 cells was capable of supporting the formation of a small number of colonies of 340A FDPC in agar (Table 5), and sustaining the viability of 340A FDPC in liquid culture (Figure 2), suggesting the possibility of autocrine production of an interleukin-3 like activity.

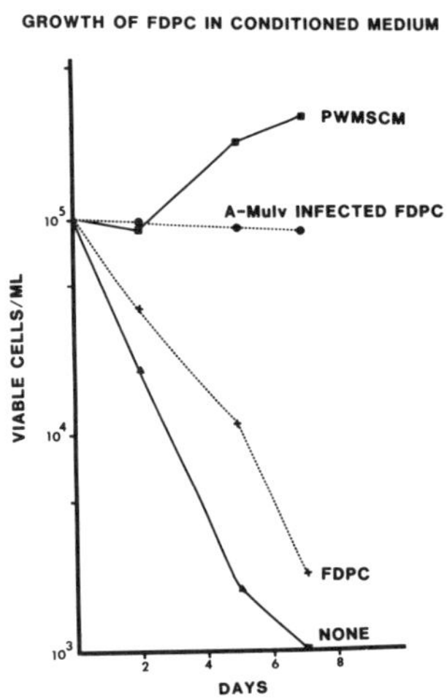

Figure 2. Growth of FDPC in 10% v/v conditioned medium from pokeweed mitogen stimulated spleen cells (PWMSCM), growth factor independent A-MuLV infected 340A-1 FDPC, and FDPC 340A.

The report of production and release of type alpha transforming growth factor (TGF) by A-MuLV transformed fibroblasts (22) prompted us to determine if A-MuLV producing FDPC produced TGF's. TGF's are low molecular weight proteins that reversibly induce cells to lose contact inhibition and undergo anchorage-independent growth *in vitro* (23). At least two types of TGF's have been identified. Type alpha TGF's, originally detected in the conditioned medium of sarcoma virus transformed cells (23), are single chain polypeptides (Mr ~6,000) that compete for binding to epidermal growth factor (EGF) receptor and have mitogenic activity (23). Type beta TGF's, present in normal as well as transformed cells (24), have neither a structural nor a functional relationship to EGF but rather modulate the level of EGF receptor, and thereby act synergistically with EGF or alpha-TGF's to induce anchorage-independent growth (25).

Serum-free CM was prepared by culture of 340A-1 cells for 48 hours at $5x10^5$ cells/ml in only RPMI 1640 medium. This serum free 340A-1 CM was compared to CM from FDPC cultured for 48 hours at $5x10^5$ cells/ml in medium supplemented with 10% PWMSCM. Neither serum free 340-1 CM nor FDPC CM was able to induce colony formation of clone 49F NRK fibroblasts in 0.3% agar between concentrations of 0.5%-40%. However, in the presence of 2 ng/ml of EGF a dose dependent increase in both the number and size of NRK colonies was seen with CM from the virus infected 340A-1 cells, but not with CM from FDPC (Figure 3). The low level of colony formation seen with FDPC CM was not statistically different than that observed with medium controls, and probably reflected the presence of EGF within the 10% fetal bovine serum, 15% horse serum, and 10% PWMSCM in this medium. These results indicated the <u>in vitro</u> A-MuLV-infected, factor independent cells were producing a beta-type TGF.

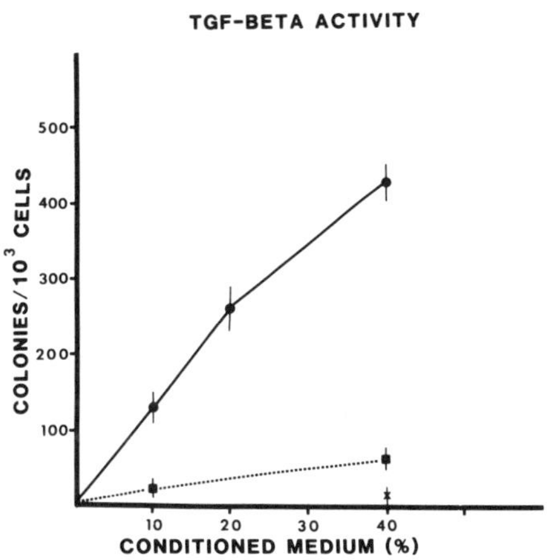

Figure 3. Stimulation of 49F NRK fibroblast colony formation in soft agar in the presence of 2 ng/ml epidermal growth factor (EGF) by conditioned medium (CM) from A-MuLV infected growth factor independent FDPC 340A-1 (——); factor dependent FDPC, 340A (---); (X) 40% 340A-1 CM without EGF.

4. DISCUSSION

Investigation of the cellular and molecular mechanisms of leukemogenesis would be facilitated by the availability of *in vitro* methods for reproducing the transforming event(s) which lead to the production of leukemic cells similar to those produced by the same leukemogen *in vivo*. Autonomous replicating promonocytic leukemia cell lines were isolated from A-MuLV leukemic mice, and found to be heterogeneous in their capacity to differentiate *in vitro* in response to GM-CSF. However, differentiated progeny of the A-MuLV leukemic cells had a reduced replicative capacity both *in vitro* and *in vivo*. In an attempt to determine if similar promonocytic leukemia lines could be generated *in vitro*, interleukin-3 growth factor dependent cells, derived from long term bone marrow cultures, were infected with A-MuLV. Growth factor independent cells could be identified within one week after A-MuLV infection, but unlike the autonomous cell lines derived from leukemic mice, these lines were poorly tumorigenic *in vivo*. Clearly, for these cells, *in vitro* induction of growth factor autonomy, following infection with A-MuLV, was not sufficient for expression of *in vivo* tumorigenicity.

Other studies of *in vitro* retrovirus infection of bone marrow culture derived cells have indicated a period of several weeks to months was often necessary before the appearance of autonomously replicating cells, and full expression of tumorigenicity (26-28). This was found both with viruses having no identifiable oncogene, the induction of erythroleukemia by a polycythemia inducing strain of spleen focus forming virus (26) and the multistep transformation of myeloblasts by Friend virus (28), and with virus with an oncogene, A-MuLV transformation of preB-lymphocytes (27).

Some of the A-MuLV infected FDPC cells in this study have been passaged weekly in interleukin-3 free medium for over 9 months (340A-1 cells) but are not able to grow progressively *in vivo* when inoculated subcutaneously, intravenously, or intraperitoneally into syngeneic mice. The reasons for the failure of these cells to grow *in vivo* is not known. They are productively infected with A-MuLV, and virus derived from these cells is fully capable of transforming fibroblasts *in vitro*. While the possible involvement of an immune response to the infected FDPC, as an explanation of their failure to grow *in vivo*, has not been directly tested, the infected FDPC produce less infectious A-MuLV and RF helper virus, and express less viral related antigens than do the highly tumorigenic AC5 and AC8 *in vivo* transformed cell lines (D.L. Hines, unpublished observations).

The loss of growth-factor dependency by the A-MuLV infected FDPC was accompanied by the appearance in the medium of growth stimulating activity for several cell types. Conditioned medium from 340A-1 cells contained GM-CSF activity, interleukin-3 like activity, and EGF potentiated transforming growth factor activity for fibroblasts. Although the actual role of these factors or activities in the loss of growth factor dependency is presently unknown, the appearance of interleukin-3 like activity suggests the loss of factor dependency may be due to the induction of autocrine production of necessary growth factors following A-MuLV infection. The development of autocrine production of growth factors as a step proceeding the development of *in vivo* tumorigenicity has been reported for the *in vitro* transformation of myeloblasts by Friend virus (21). Thus, it is possible the growth factor independent FDPC will eventually develop *in vivo* tumorigenicity, but to date this particular system has not been useful for studying the progression of leukemic potential.

This paper also describes clonal variation in capacity for differentiation among promonocytic leukemic cell lines derived from individual leukemic animals. None of 25 clonal lines required an exogenous source of GM-CSF for growth *in vitro*, however they differed significantly in the production of differentiated progeny when cultured with GM-CSF. Seventeen lines produced an increased proportion of colonies containing differentiated cells when cultured in agar in the presence of GM-CSF, 5 lines did not, and 3 lines never produced differentiated cells. Recognition of the heterogenity in the responsiveness of leukemic stem cells derived from the same leukemia is important in considering induction of differentiation as a therapeutic approach to the treatment of myelogenous leukemia (29). However, it is significant that in these retrovirus transformed leukemic cells, differentiation was accompanied by a reduction in proliferative capacity both *in vitro* and *in vivo*. Studies determining the effect of differentiation on expression of viral genes are in progress.

ACKNOWLEDGMENT

This work was supported by Public Health Service grants CA 25234 and CA25391 from the National Cancer Institute, by the E. Walter Albacten Bequest, and an Institutional Grant to the Michigan Cancer Foundation from the United Foundation of Greater Detroit.

REFERENCES

1. Foulds L: The experimental study of tumor progression: A review. Cancer Res. 14:327-339, 1954.
2. Fialkow PJ: Cell lineages in hematopoietic neoplasia studied with glycose-6-phosphate dehydrogenase cell markers. J. Cell Physiol. Suppl. 1:37-43, 1982.
3. McCulloch EA: Stem cells in normal and leukemic hemopoiesis. Blood 62:1-13, 1983.
4. Park CH, Amare M, Savin MA, Goodwin JW, Newcomb MM, Hoogstraten B: Prediction of chemotherapy response in human leukemia using an *in vitro* chemotherapy sensitivity test on the leukemic colony-forming cells. Blood 55:595-601, 1980.
5. Boggs DR: Hematopoietic stem cell theory in relation to possible lymphoblastic conversion of chronic myeloid leukemia. Blood 44:449-453, 1974.

6. Dexter TM, Testa NG: Differentiation and proliferation of hemopoietic cells in culture. Meth. Cell Biol. 14:387-405, 1976.
7. Dexter TM, Allen TD, Lajtha LJ: Conditions controling the proliferation of haemopoietic stem cells *in vitro*. J. Cell Physiol. 91:335-349, 1977.
8. Greenberger JS, Davisson PB, Gans PJ, Moloney WC: *In vitro* induction of continuous acute promyelocytic leukemia cell lines by Friend or Abelson murine leukemia virus. Blood 53:987-1001, 1979.
9. Dexter TM, Garland J, Scott D, Scolnick E, Metcalf D: Growth of factor-dependent hemopoietic precursor cell lines. J. Exp. Med. 152:1036-1097, 1980.
10. Greenberger JS, Eckner RJ, Sakakeeny M, Marks P, Reid D, Nabel G, Hapel A, Ihle JN, Humphries KC: Interleukin 3-dependent hematopoietic progenitor cell lines. Federation Proc. 42:2762-2771, 1983.
11. Schrader JW: Bone marrow differentiation *in vitro*. CRC Crit. Rev. Immunol. 4:197-277, 1983.
12. Greenberger JS, Sakakeeny MA, Humphries RK, Eaves CJ, Eckner RJ: Demonstration of permanent factor-dependent multipotential (erythroid/neutrophil/basophil) hematopoietic progenitor cell lines. Proc. Natl. Sci. USA 80: 2931-2935, 1983.
13. Reddy EP, Smith MJ, Srinivassan A: Nucleotide sequence of Abelson murine leukemia virus genome: Structural similarity of its transforming gene product to other onc gene products with tyrosine-specific kinase activity. Proc. Natl. Acad. Sci. USA 80:3623-3627, 1983.
14. Witte ON, Dasgorpta A, Baltimore D: Abelson murine leukemia virus protein is phosphorylated *in vitro* to form phosphotyrosine. Nature (London) 283:826-831, 1980.
15. Rosenberg N, Baltimore D: A quantitative assay for transformation of bone marrow cells by Abelson murine leukemia virus. J. Exp. Med. 143:1453-1463, 1976.
16. Rosenberg N, Baltimore D: Abelson Virus. In: Viral Oncology, Klein G (ed), (New York, Raven Press), 1980, pp. 187-203.
17. Hines DL, Gragowski L: Abelson murine leukemia virus: Effect of helper virus from regressing Friend virus on leukemia development. Leuk. Res. 7:251-260, 1983.
18. Raschke WC, Baird S, Ralph P, Nakoinz I: Functional macrophage cell lines transformed by Abelson leukemia virus. Cell 15:261-267, 1978.
19. Hines DL: Lipid accumulation and production of colony-stimulating activity by the 266AD cell line derived from mouse bone marrow. Blood 61:397-402, 1983.
20. Brennan JK, Abboud CN, DiPersio JF, Barlow GH, Lichtman MA: Autostimulation of growth by human myelogenous leukemia cells (HL-60). Blood 58:803-812, 1981.
21. Heard JM, Fichelson S, Choppin J, Varet B: Autocrine function of murine F-MuLV induced myeloblastic cell lines. Int. J. Cancer 31:337-344, 1983.

22. Twardzik DR, Todaro GJ, Marquardt H, Reynolds FH, Stephenson JR: Transformation induced by Abelson murine leukemia virus involves production of a polypeptide growth factor. Science 216:894-897, 1982.
23. Delarco J, Todaro G: Growth factors from murine sarcoma virus-transformed cells. Proc. Natl. Acad. Sci. USA 75: 4001-4005, 1978.
24. Assoian R, Komoriya A, Myers C, Spron M: Transforming growth factor-B in human platelets: Indentification of a major storage site, purification and characterization. J. Biol. Chem. 258:7155-7160, 1983.
25. Assoian R, Frolik CA, Roberts AB, Miller DM, Spron MB: Transforming growth factor-B controls receptor levels for epidermal growth factor in NRK fibroblasts. Cell 36:35-41, 1984.
26. Dexter TM, Allen TD, Testa NG, Scolnick E: Friend disease in vitro. J. Exp. Med. 154:594-608, 1981.
27. Whitlock CA, Ziegler SF, Witte ON: Progression of the transformed phenotype in clonal lines of Abelson virus-infected lymphocytes. Mol. and Cell Bio. 3:596-604, 1983.
28. Heard JM, Fichelson S, Sola B, Martial MA, Berger R, Varet B, Levy JP: Malignant myeloblastic transformation of murine long-term bone-marrow cultures by F-MuLV: In vitro reproduction of a long-term leukemogenesis and investigation of preleukemic events. Int. J. Cancer 32:237-245, 1983.
29. Koeffler HP: Induction of differentiation of human acute myelogenous leukemia cells: Therapeutic implications. Blood 62:709-721, 1983.

7

CHEMOTHERAPEUTIC AGENTS AS DIFFERENTIATION INDUCERS

Dr. Alexander Bloch

Almost all clinically effective anticancer agents are inhibitors of DNA synthesis or transcription (1). Inhibitors that interfere with RNA or protein synthesis or with the metabolism of other cell components lack selective antitumor activity. If cytotoxicity, which forms the basis for current treatment regimens, were the major determinant for selective antitumor action, then inhibitors of cellular targets other than DNA should have emerged as clinically effective agents. Since that is not the case, selective antitumor action would appear to depend on the inhibition of DNA-centered activities that relate to the maintenance of tumor cell growth.

Neoplastic cells are characterized by their arrest at stages of immature differentiation, but they retain their capacity for unrestricted proliferation (2,3). Because of this imbalance, a population of immature cells emerges that gives rise to the clinical entity we call "cancer". If the maturation-arrested cancer cells could be induced to differentiate to more advanced maturation stages, at which they become again sensitive to normal growth and differentiation controls, or to terminally mature non-proliferating cells, a tangible therapeutic benefit would likely result.

Experimental evidence has been adduced which suggests that the antitumor-selective action of the DNA-specific agents derives from their ability to initiate maturation events (4). For example, at minimally- or non-toxic concentrations, clinically effective DNA-specific agents such as daunorubicin, araC, and

6-mercaptopurine are capable of inducing the differentiation of human myeloblastic leukemia cells (ML-1) to monocyte/macrophages (5). Agents such as cordycepin or α-amanitin which interfere with RNA synthesis, or puromycin and cycloheximide which inhibit protein synthesis are unable to induce these maturation events (4). Interference with DNA synthesis or transcription at non- or minimally cytotoxic concentrations of DNA-specific agents impedes transcription of the actively ongoing proliferation program of the cancer cell, leading to the subsequent expression of genetic information that determines cell maturation (Fig. 1).

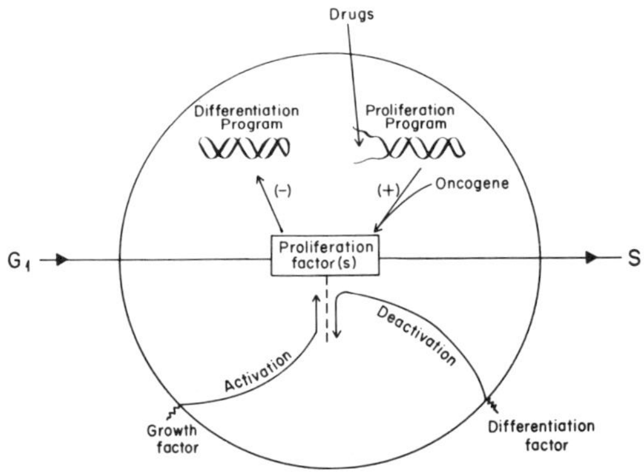

Figure 1.

Since RNA and protein synthesis are required for proliferation of the cancer cell as well as for its maturation, agents that interfere with the metabolism of these macromolecules are unable to induce differentiation. Inhibitors of RNA and protein synthesis can interfere with tumor cell growth only at cytotoxic concentrations that preclude antitumor selectivity.

The ability of DNA-specific agents to induce cancer cell maturation at marginally toxic doses depends, however, on the presence of natural differentiation factors (DF). These are present in the hemopoietic microenvironment, and are supplied to the cells in culture by the fetal serum. Leukemic cells, analogous to their normal counterparts, respond to both growth and differentiation factors (6-8), but their sensitivity to these opposing controls appears to have shifted in favor of the growth signal. That does not mean that cancer cells have lost their ability to respond to stimulation by DF. An increase in the concentration of natural DF above the level present in serum leads to the ready differentiation of the leukemic cells (8,9). By interfering with the expression of proliferation-associated information, the DNA-targeted agents increase the sensitivity of the leukemic cell to the action of DF, so that differentiation occurs at a concentration of DF that would not normally suffice for initiating maturation (10,11). This sensitization phenomenon can be explained by postulating the existence of a labile intracellular proliferation protein that, at a sufficiently high concentration, causes cell cycle transit from G_1 to S (12). Its concentration in the cell is controlled in an inverse manner by DF and GF, low concentrations of GF or elevated levels of DF (13) leading to its decay, followed by activation of the differentiation path. Lowering the level of the DNA transcript that specifies the proliferation protein by exposing the cells to DNA-reactive agents, augments the DF signal causing differentiation. It is likely that this phenomenon of "sensitization" constitutes a critical component of successful clinical drug therapy. Because sensitization occurs at low drug concentrations, this concept provides a rational basis for the use of low-dose regimens that cause little, if any, host toxicity.

Since initiation of differentiation by the DNA-targeted drugs depends on the availability of DF, the concentration at which these factors are present in the individual to be treated is a major determinant of therapeutic outcome. If factor production is low, non-cytotoxic drug regimens will not likely lead to an effective response. Under such circumstances, pharmaceutical preparations of DF would offer a potentially useful remedy. Since the concentration of constitutive DF for hemopoietic cells is generally low and their elaboration likely restricted to the microenvironment of the bone marrow, DNA recombinant techniques may be most suitable for their production in quantities sufficient for therapeutic use. Since various polymers such as poly (I).poly (C) (14), certain corticosteroids including dexamethasone and prednisolone (15), and various immunostimulating bacterial extracts such as BCG (16) are capable of enhancing the formation of DF by producer cells, use of these agents in conjunction with DNA-specific inhibitors offers an additional opportunity for improving therapeutic outcome.

The growth of a majority of tumor cell lines remains dependent upon the presence of GF provided by the serum. Agents that prevent the binding of these factors to specific cell receptors or that interfere with the transmission of the growth signal enhance the transition from proliferation to differentiation. Among such agents are certain phorbol esters (17) and retinoic acid (18). Polar substances such as dimethyl sulfoxide (5,19, 20) likely induce differentiation by non-specifically modifying receptor sensitivity through their interaction with the lipid membrane.

The ability to induce tumor cell maturation by these modalities demonstrates that the oncogenic arrest of normal cell differentiation is not necessarily an irrevocable event. What is required for reversion to the normal state is the specific interruption of molecular events that freeze the cancer cell in its proliferation mode. Cellular oncogene products play a crucial role in establishing this freeze, possibly through their structural or functional relationship to natural GF or to protein kinases regulated by GF (21-25). Whatever the case, the initiation of leukemic cell differentiation by any of the synthetic or natural inducers results in the very rapid decline of pertinent oncogene transcripts (26).

From the clinical point of view, the differentiation-centered approach allows the use of regimens that are minimally- or non-toxic. Since the demonstrated sensitization of leukemic cells by DNA-reactive agents occurs at non-cytotoxic concentrations, low-dose regimens should theoretically suffice to bring about a therapeutic response. In fact, such regimens have demonstrated significant therapeutic activity in various initial clinical trials (27-31). Since the effectiveness of low drug doses would appear to depend upon adequate levels of DF, the availability of these factors in the patient is a critical component of successful treatment.

Where DF concentrations are inadequate, the therapeutic response to low-dose regimens with DNA-targeted agents is likely to be minimal. Under such circumstances, the administration of exogenous preparations of DF or of agents that stimulate DF formation by producer cells would likely improve the therapeutic outcome. DF are produced by more mature cells within the hematopoietic system to which the leukemic cell belongs (32-34). Since tumor cells, analogous to their normal counterparts, elaborate factors that can inhibit stem- and precursor cell renewal (35,36), mature cells are prevented from emerging, and removal of the tumor cell burden aids the reestablishment of factor-centered control. Once conversion of the tumor cells to more mature forms has occurred, they are again capable of producing appropriate factors (37).

The means to be employed for reducing the tumor burden depends upon the prevailing level of DF. If that level is too low, large-scale induction of tumor cell differentiation by non-toxic concentrations of DNA-reactive drugs cannot be expected to occur. Other remedies become then necessary. These include the parenteral administration of DF, once these become available in quantity, or the removal of a significant portion of the cancer cell population by cytolytic hormones or by inhibitors of GF binding or signalling. Regimens that rely upon maximally tolerated cytotoxicity may be counterproductive, since they are likely to suppress the emergence of normal cells that are required for factor production. Where frankly cytotoxic regimens have proved effective, drug levels reached in the marrow may have been low enough to allow sensitization of the tumor cells to the DF signal without destroying the stem cell population. In fact, it would appear permissible to remove a significant portion of the systemic tumor cell population by cytotoxic means, if such treatment preserves the factor-producing elements.

Since solid tumors can also be viewed as originating from arrested cell maturation (38,39), the same therapeutic principles as outlined for the leukemias apply. Various clinically responsive solid tumors respond to *in vitro* drug treatment by initiating differentiation (40-43). The major obstacle to a maturation-based approach derives from the low cycling fraction that characterizes solid tumors such as the colo-rectal carcinomas (44). This limitation requires that a drug be applied over prolonged periods of time, or that GF be provided simultaneously with DF. Recruiting the non-cycling fraction into growth, renders it susceptible to the action of DF.

By employing such modalities, the maturation-centered approach would appear to hold tangible promise for improving the therapy of cancer.

ACKNOWLEDGEMENT

The studies cited in this paper were supported in part by Public Health Service, DHHS, grant CA-36241 from the National Cancer Institute.

REFERENCES

1. Bloch A: Purine and pyrimidine analogs in cancer chemotherapy. In: New Leads in Cancer Therapeutics, Mihich E (ed), Boston, GK Hall and Co., 1981, pp. 65-72.

2. Pierce G, Shiles R, Fink L: Cancer, a problem of developmental biology. Englewood Cliffs, Prentice Hall, 1978.
3. Greaves MP: "Target" cells, cellular phenotypes, and lineage fidelity in human leukemia. J. Cell Physiol. Suppl. 1:113-125, 1982.
4. Takeda K, Minowada J, Leasure JA, Bloch A: Comparison of the ability of various cytotoxic agents to induce the differentiation of human myeloblastic leukemia cells _in vitro_. Proc. Am. Assoc. Cancer Res. 23:226, 1982.
5. Takeda K, Minowada J, Bloch A: Kinetics of appearance of differentiation-associated characteristics in ML-1, a line of human myeloblastic leukemia cells, after treatment with 12-0-tetradecanoylphorbol-13-acetate, dimethyl sulfoxide, or 1-B-D-arabinofuranosylcytosine. Cancer Research 42: 5152-5158, 1982.
6. Maeda M, Ichikava Y: Production of growth and differentiation-stimulating factors for mouse leukemia cells by different cell species. Gann 64:257-263, 1973.
7. Yamamoto Y, Tomida M, Hozumi M: Production by mouse spleen cells of factors stimulating differentiation of mouse myeloid leukemic cells that differ from the colony-stimulating factor. Cancer Res. 40:4804-4809, 1980.
8. Takeda K, Minowada J, Bloch A: Differential ability of mitogen-stimulated human leukocyte-conditioned media to induce F_C receptors in human leukemia cells. Cell Immunol. 79:288-297, 1983.
9. Craig RW, Frankfurt O, Sakagami H, Takeda K, Bloch A: Macromolecular and cell cycle effects of different classes of agents inducing the maturation of human myeloblastic leukemia (ML-1) cells. Cancer Res. 44:2421-2429, 1984.
10. Hayashi M, Okabe J, Hozumi M: Sensitization of resistant myeloid leukemia cells by anticancer drugs to factor-stimulating differentiation. Gann 70:235-238, 1979.
11. Okabe J, Honma Y, Hayashi M, Hozumi M: Actinomycin D restores _in vivo_ sensitivity to differentiation induction of non-differentiating mouse myeloid leukemia cells. Int. J. Cancer 24:87-91, 1979.
12. Medrano EE, Aranyi P, Pardee AB: On the regulation of eukaryotic cell growth: An approach to the behavior of normal and transformed cells. In: Cellular Responses to Molecular Modulators. Mozes LW, Schultz J, Scott WP, Warner R (eds), New York, Academic Press, 1981, pp. 49-51.
13. Ballard FJ, Knowles SE, Wong SC, Bodner JB, Wood CM, Gunn JM: Inhibition of protein breakdown in cultured cells is a consistent response to growth factors. FEBS Lett 144:209-212, 1980.
14. Tomida M, Yamamoto Y, Hozumi M: Inhibition of leukemogenicity of myeloid leukemic cells in mice and _in vivo_ induction of normal differentiation of the cells by poly(I).poly(C). Gann 71:457-463, 1980.

15. Honma V, Kasukabe T, Hozumi M: Production of differentiation-stimulating factor in cultured mouse myeloid leukemia cells treated by glucocorticoids. Expt. Cell Res. 111:261-267, 1978.
16. Yamamoto Y, Tomida M, Hozumi M et al: Enhancement by immunostimulants of the production by mouse spleen cells of factor(s) stimulating differentiation of mouse myeloid leukemic cells. Gann 72:828-833, 1981.
17. Lee L-S, Weinstein IB: Tumor-promoting phorbol esters inhibit binding of epidermal growth factor to cellular receptors. Science 202:314-315, 1978.
18. Jetten AM: Effects of retinoic acid on the binding and mitogenic activity of epidermal growth factor. J. Cell Physiol. 110:235-240, 1982.
19. Friend C, Scher W, Holland JG, Sato T: Hemoglobin synthesis in murine virus induced leukemic cells <u>in vitro</u>: Stimulation of erythoid differentiation by dimethyl sulfoxide. Proc. Nat. Acad. Sci. (USA) 68:378-382, 1971.
20. Collins SJ, Ruscetti FW, Gallagher RE, Gallo RC: Terminal differentiation of human promyelocytic leukemia cells induced by dimethylsulfoxide and other polar compounds. Proc. Natl. Acad. Sci. (USA) 75:2458-2462, 1980.
21. Todaro GJ, DeLarco JE, Cohen S: Transformation by murine and feline sarcomas viruses specifically blocks binding of epidermal growth factor to cells. Nature 264:26-31, 1976.
22. Cohen S, Carpenter G, King L Jr: Epidermal growth factor-receptor-protein kinase interactions. J. Biol. Chem. 255:4834-4842, 1980.
23. Ushiro H, Cohen S: Identification of phosphotyrosine as a product of epidermal growth factor-activated protein kinase in A-431 cell membrane. J. Biol. Chem. 255:8363-8365, 1980.
24. Kudlow JE, Buss JE, Gill GN: Anit-pp60^{src} antibodies are substrates for EGF-stimulated protein kinase. Nature 290:519-521, 1981.
25. Doolittle RF, Hunkapiller MW, Aaronson SA, Antoniades HN: Simian sarcoma virus onc gene, v-sis, is derived from the gene (or genes) encoding a platelet-derived growth factor. Science 221:275-277, 1983.
26. Craig RW, Bloch A: Expression of a cellular oncogene (myb) declines early in induced myeloblastic leukemia cell differentiation. Cancer Res. 44:442-446, 1984.
27. Baccarani M, Tura S: Differentiation of myeloid leukemic cells: New possibilities for therapy. Br. J. Haematol. 42:485-490, 1979.
28. Housett M, Daniel MT, Degos L: Small doses of ara-C in the treatment of acute myeloid leukemia: Differentiation of myeloid leukemia cells. Br. J. Haematol. 51:125-129, 1982.
29. Maloney WC, Rosenthal DS: Treatment of early acute nonlymphatic leukemia with low dose cytosine arabinoside. In: Modern Trends in Human Leukemia. Neth, Gallo RC, Graf T et al (eds), pp. 59-62, Springer, Berlin.

30. Schiff RD, Mertelsmann R, Andreeff M, Gee TS, Kempin SJ, Koziner BL, Lee BJ and Clarkson BD: Low-dose arabinosyl cytosine (LD ARA-C) In: Hematologic Malignancies and Myelodysplastic Syndromes (MDS). Proceedings Amer. Soc. Clin. Onc. 3:206, 1984.
31. Griffin J, Wisch J, Kufe D: Lose dose ARA-C therapy in preleukemic syndromes. Proceedings Amer. Soc. Clin. Onc. 3:195, 1984.
32. Clarkson B, Marks PA, Till JE: Differentiation of normal and neoplastic hematopoietic cells. Cold Spring Harbor Laboratory, 1978.
33. Mak TW, McCullough EA: Cellular and molecular biology of hemopoietic stem cell differentiation. New York, AR Liss, 1982.
34. Sachs L: Control of growth and normal differentiation in leukemia cells: Regulation of the developmental program and restoration of the normal phenotype in myeloid leukemia. J. Cell Physiol. Supp. 1:151-164, 1982.
35. Okabe J, Hayashi M, Honma Y, Hozumi M: Differentiation of mouse myeloid leukemia cells is inhibited by a factor from non-differentiating leukemia cells. Intl. J. Cancer 22: 570-575, 1978.
36. Broxmeyer HE, Jacobsen N, Kurland J, Mendelsohn N, Moore MAS: In vitro suppression of normal granulocytic stem cells by inhibitory activity derived from human leukemia cells. J. Natl. Cancer Inst. 60:497-510, 1978.
37. Maeda M, Ichikawa Y: Production of a colony-stimulating factor following differentiation of leukemia myeloblasts to macrophages. J. Cell Physiol. 102:323-331, 1980.
38. Lipkin M: Proliferation and differentiation of gastrointestinal cells in normal and disease states. In: Physiology of the Gastrointestinal Tract. Johnson L (ed), New York, Raven Press, 1981, pp. 145-167.
39. Lipkin M, Blattner WE, Fraumeini J Jr, Lynch HT, Dreschner E, Winawer S: Tritiated thymidine labeling distribution as a marker for hereditary predisposition to colon cancer. Cancer Res. 43:1899-1904, 1983.
40. Schubert D, Jacob F: 5-bromodeoxyuridine-induced differentiation of a neuroblastoma. Proc. Natl. Acad. Sci. (USA) 67:247-254, 1970.
41. Silbert SW, Goldstein MN: Drug-induced differentiation of a rat glioma in vitro. Cancer Res. 32:1422-1427, 1972.
42. Friedman SJ, Skehan P: Morphological differentiation of human choriocarcinoma cells induced by methotrexate. Cancer Res. 39:1960-1967, 1979.
43. Strickland S, Sawey MJ: Studies on the effect of retinoids on the differentiation of teratocarcinoma stem cells in vitro and in vivo. Developmental Biol. 78:76-85, 1980.
44. Weisburger JH, Reddy BS, Joftes DL: Colo-rectal cancer report no. 19. Intl. Union Against Cancer, Geneva, pp. 69-76, 1975.

8

MODES OF DRUG RESISTANCE IN ACUTE LEUKEMIAS

Dr. David Kessel

This article provides a brief overview of mechanisms whereby acute leukemias become drug resistant. Modes of resistance to methotrexate and cytosine arabinoside are briefly summarized. Recent information on resistance to the natural products (vinca alkaloids, anthracyclines) is described in more detail.

1. INTRODUCTION

Examples of drug resistance have been observed with every new anti-neoplastic agent. The topic has been the subject of recent reviews (1-5) which have described the various mechanisms whereby drug responsiveness is altered. These can be divided into three general classes.

1. Drug resistance related to exposure of predominantly non-dividing cells to agents which exert their major cytotoxic activity in the S phase of the cell cycle.
2. Resistance associated with appearance of tumor cells in a body compartment not accessible to circulating drug.
3. Resistance resulting from mutational events. These include loss of capacity for drug accumulation, loss of drug-activating enzymes, enhanced repair of drug-induced damage.

An understanding of modes of drug resistance can lead to development of improved anti-tumor agents, and more effective scheduling programs. Procedures for the circumvention of drug resistance can be devised once modes of resistance are understood. The increasing use of combination drug therapy has, in part, resulted from an understanding of the need for agents active against both proliferating and non-proliferating cell populations, together with the need for rapid eradication of a neoplastic cell population before multi-drug resistance clones can arise.

2. METHOTREXATE RESISTANCE

Methotrexate was among the earliest agents to be effectively employed in the treatment of acute leukemia in children. The major modes of drug resistance include elevated levels of the target enzyme, dihydrofolate reductase, loss of a system which mediates drug uptake, and reduced formation of intracellular methotrexate polyglutamates (2,6,7). Elevated levels of the target enzyme have been associated with a phenomenon called gene amplification (8), wherein a large number of copies of the gene sequence coding for dihydrofolate reductase are found in drug-resistant cells. A lack of understanding of these modes of drug resistance can be fatal to drug development strategies. For example, a methotrexate analog which inactivated tumor cell but not liver dihydrofolate reductase was developed by Baker et al. in 1969 (9), but the drug was not able to penetrate cell membranes and was therefore inactive.

3. CYTOSINE ARABINOSIDE

We had initially shown that resistance to this agent, in acute and chronic leukemias, was associated with impaired drug phosphorylation (10). Elevated pools of dCTP have also been implicated in examples of drug resistance in cell culture (11). In a study of marrow and peripheral neoplastic cells from leukemia patients and normal donors, no correlation could be found between rates of drug phosphorylation and araCTP retention vs. cytotoxicity *in vitro* (12). But araCTP retention had previously been correlated with drug responsiveness *in vivo* (13). In another report, responsiveness to cytosine arabinoside was found correlated with rates of mediated drug influx *in vitro* (14). Since both impaired uptake and impaired phosphorylation have been identified as modes of drug resistance, clinical trials of high-dose cytosine arabinoside were devised (15,16), with some reported successes in leukemias refractory to conventional drug therapy.

4. ANTHRACYCLINE AND VINCRISTINE RESISTANCE

Resistance to these natural products, in cell culture, has been associated with an outward drug transport process which serves to limit intracellular drug concentration to sub-lethal levels (17). It has recently been shown that this mode of drug resistance can be circumvented by a series of agents classified as calcium antagonists (18-21). Although the mode of action of these agents was initially believed to involve effects on calcium fluxes, we have established different modes of action (22). The calcium antagonist verapamil is effective at 3-5 uM extracellular levels, and acts as a competitive inhibitor of the outward anthracycline transport system. In contrast, nifedipine and its analogs are effective at high intracellular levels, perhaps via a chaotropic process resulting in membrane disruption. Use of calcium + anthracyclines might result in circumvention of resistance to adriamycin and daunorubicin in acute leukemias, if results from the animal tumor trials could be translated into clinical successes. Moreover, combined treatment with tocopherol + nifedipine was found to protect cancer patients from adverse effects of adriamycin to the heart (23). Unfortunately, verapamil increased cardiotoxicity of adriamycin to the rabbit heart (24).

Our studies on 13 patients with acute myelocytic leukemia varying widely in adriamycin responsiveness were not encouraging (25). The uptake of labeled drug *in vitro* was not correlated with subsequent adriamycin responsiveness *in vivo*, nor could we find any evidence for the presence of an outward drug transport process in myeloblasts obtained from patients with adriamycin-refractory leukemias. In another series of studies, we were not able to demonstrate impaired anthracycline accumulation in a series of solid murine tumors never grown in culture (26). The enhanced exodus system may therefore be relevant in examples of resistance to anthracyclines and other natural products only in cell culture, where cells can be selected for resistance to clinically-unattainable drug levels.

Examples of resistance to the natural products, in cell culture, has also been associated with the appearance of new membrane glycoprotein with a molecular weight of approximately 200,000 Daltons (27,28). Enhanced phosphorylation of a membrane glycoprotein was also found when drug-resistant cells were exposed to metabolic inhibitors (29). In a related study, Beck (30) reported that the enhanced exodus of vinca alkaloids from a drug-resistant cell line was related to an energy-dependent binding phenomenon. Beck postulated that the drug-resistant cell contained drug binding sites which were inactivated by an energy-dependent process. In this model, the enhanced drug exodus from resistant cells is based on the failure of a binding process, rather than an outward transport system. The finding by Center (29) that membrane glycoprotein phosphorylation is enhanced under conditions (presence of metabolic inhibitors) which promote drug retention by resistant cells provides support for Beck's model. But this model does not explain the ability of a non-toxic anthracycline analog (31) to promote daunorubicin accumulation; competition for exodus would appear to be a more likely explanation.

All of the studies cited above, where drug resistance was associated with both new membrane glycoprotein species and membrane protein phosphorylation, involved highly drug-resistant cell lines maintained in culture. In studies on spontaneous and drug-induced murine solid tumors, we found no evidence for the presence of resistance-associated membrane glycoprotein species, nor could such components be identified in membranes of freshly-isolated circulating myeloblasts from patients with anthracycline-resistant acute leukemias (26).

5. SUMMARY

The study of modes of drug resistance has provided a substantial amount of evidence that tumor cells can escape the toxicity of conventional chemotherapy. Unfortunately, the normal cells of the host lack such escape mechanisms. Drug resistance can be circumvented by a variety of means, including drug combinations, high-dose regimens, and use of second agents to modify resistance patterns.

It is tempting to speculate that newer modalities, e.g., the biologic response modifiers, may mediate tumor cell eradication via mechanisms to which resistance cannot occur. But as such modalities receive more attention, it is also possible that new modes of resistance will arise, challenging our imagination for the generation of new concepts in resistance circumvention.

ACKNOWLEDGMENT

The research from our laboratory described here was supported by grants CA 31331, CA 16053, CA 11242 and contract PH 43-66-541 from the National Cancer Institute, NIH, DHHS.

REFERENCES

1. Cheng Y-C, Brockman RW: Mechanisms of drug resistance and collateral sensitivity: basis for development of chemotherapeutic agents. In: Development of Target-Oriented Anticancer Drugs, Cheng YC et al (eds), Raven Press, New York, 1983, pp. 107-117.
2. Bertino JR, Srimatkandada S, Carman MD, Schornagel JH, Medina WD, Moroson BA, Cashmore AR, Weiner HL, Dube SK: Mechanisms of Methotrexate resistance in acute leukemia. In: Normal and Neoplastic Hematopoiesis, Alan R. Liss, NY, 1983, pp. 465-478.
3. Skipper HE, Schabel FM Jr.: Tumor stem cell heterogeneity: implications with respect to classification of cancers by chemotherapeutic effect. Cancer Treatment Repts. 68:43-61, 1984.
4. Curt GA, Clendeninn NJ, Chabner BA: Drug resistance in cancer. Cancer Treatment Repts. 68:87-99, 1984.
5. Symposium on cellular resistance to anticancer drugs. Cancer Treatment Repts. 67:855-932, 1983.

6. Jolivet J, Cowan KH, Curt GA, Clendininn NJ, Chabner BA: The pharmacology and clinical use of methotrexate. New Eng. J. Med. 309:1094-1104, 1983.
7. Rosenblatt DS, Whitehead VM: Methotrexate polyglutamates in cultured human cells. In: Folyl and Antifolyl Polyglutamates. Goldman ID, Chabner BA, Bertino Jr. (eds), Plenum Press, 1983, pp. 275-285.
8. Schimke RA, Kaufman RJ, Alt FW, Kellems RF: Gene amplification and drug resistance in cultured murine cells. Science 202:1051-1056, 1978.
9. Baker BR, Meyer RB Jr.: Irreversible Enzyme Inhibitors. J. Med. Chem. 12:224-227, 1969.
10. Kessel D, Hall TC, Rosenthal D: Uptake and phosphorylation of cytosine arabinoside by normal and leukemic human blood cells in vitro. Cancer Res. 29:459-463, 1969.
11. Vincent BR, Butten G: Studies on 1-B-D-arabinofuranosylcytosine resistant mutants of Chinese hamster fibroblasts. Somat. Cell Genet. 39:42-49, 1979.
12. Epstein J, Preisler HD, Rustum YM, Higby DJ: Effects of cytosine arabinoside on unseparated bone marrow and peripheral blood cells and on specimens enriched for myeloblasts and promyeloctyes. Exp. Hemat. 8:404-408, 1980.
13. Rustum YM, Preisler HD: Correlation between leukemic cell retention of 1-B-D-arabinofuranosyl cytosine 5'-triphosphate and response to therapy. Cancer Res. 39:42-49, 1979.
14. Wiley JS, Jones SP, Sawyer WH, Paterson ARP: Cytosine arabinoside influx and nucleoside transport sites in acute leukemia. J. Clin. Invest. 69:479-489, 1982.
15. Andreeff M, Kewmin S, Arlin Z, Mertelsmann R, Espiritu E, Gee T: High-dose cytosine arabinoside in acute leukemia: correlation of clinical response and cell kinetics. Proc. Amer. Assn. Cancer Res. 24:166, 1983.
16. Febres R, Flessa HC, Martelo OJ: Efficacy of high dose cytosine arabinoside in refractory adult leukemia. Proc. Amer. Soc. Clin. Onc. 1:128, 1982.
17. Danø K, Skovsgaard T, Nissen NI, Friche E, Di Marco A: Mechanism of resistance to anthracyclines and vinca alkaloids. 13th International Cancer Congress Part C, Biology of Cancer (2), Alan R. Liss, New York, 1983, pp. 231-246.
18. Slater LM, Murray SL, Wetzel MW, Wisdon RM, DuVall EM: Verapamil restoration of daunorubicin responsiveness in daunorubicin-resistant Ehrlich ascites carcinoma. J. Clin. Invest. 70:1131-1134, 1980.
19. Tsuruo T, Iida H, Tsukagoshi S, Sakurai Y: Overcoming of vincristine resistance in P388 leukemia in vivo and in vitro through enhanced cytotoxicity of vincristine and vinblastine by verapamil. Cancer Res. 41:1967-1972, 1981.
20. Tsuruo T, Iida H, Tsukagoshi S, Sakurai Y: Increased accumulation of vincristine and adriamycin in drug-resistant P388 tumor cells following incubation with calcium antagonists and calmodulin inhibitors. Cancer Res. 42:4730-4733, 1982.

21. Tsuruo T, Iida H, Yamashiro M, Tsukagoshi S, Sakurai Y: Enhancement of vincristine- and adriamycin-induced cytotoxicity by verapamil in P388 leukemia and its sublines resistant to vincristine and adriamycin. Biochem. Pharmacol. 31:3138-3140, 1982.
22. Kessel D, Wilberding C: Mode of action of calcium antagonists which alter anthracycline resistance. Biochem. Pharmacol. In Press, 1984.
23. Lenzhofer R, Ganzinger U, Rameis H, Moser K: Acute cardiac toxicity in patients after doxorubicin treatment and the effect of combined tocopherol and nifedipine treatment. J. Cancer Res. Clin. Oncol. 106:143-147, 1973.
24. Rabkin SW, Otten M, Polimeni PI: Increased mortality with cardiotoxic doses of adriamycin after verapamil pretreatpent despite prevention of myocardial calcium accumulapion. Can. J. Physiol. Pharmacol. 61:1050-1056, 1983.
25. Kessel D, Wilberding C, Ratanatharathorn V: Daunorubicin accumulation by human myeloblasts varying in anthracycline resistance. Cancer Research, In Press, 1984.
26. Kessel D, Wilberding C, Corbett T: Studies on anthracycline resistance. Proc. Amer. Assn. Cancer Res. 25:297, 1984.
27. Kartner N, Riordan JR, Ling V: Cell surface P glycoprotein associated with multi-drug resistance in mammalian cell lines. Science 221:1285-1288, 1983.
28. Beck WT, Mueller TJ, Tanzer LR: Altered surface membrane glycoproteins in vinca alkaloid-resistant human leukemic lymphoblasts. Cancer Res. 39:2070-2076, 1979.
29. Center MS: Evidence that adriamycin resistance in Chinese hamster lung cells is regulated by phosphorylation of a plasma membrane glycoprotein. Biochem. Biophys. Res. Commun. 115:159-166, 1983.
30. Beck WT, Cirtain MC, Lefko JL: Energy-dependent reduced drug binding as a mechanism of vinca alkaloid resistance in human leukemic lymphocytes. Molec. Pharmacol. 24:485-492, 1983.
31. Skovsgaard T: Circumvention of resistance to daunorubicin by N-acetyldaunorubicin in Ehrlich ascites tumor. Cancer Res. 40:1077-1083, 1980.

9

THE EVOLUTION OF THERAPY FOR ACUTE LYMPHATIC LEUKEMIA IN CHILDREN

Teresa J. Vietti, M.D. and James Boyett, Ph.D.

1. INDUCTION THERAPY - SINGLE AGENTS

In 1948, Dr. Farber and his colleagues (1) used the first effective antileukemic agent, aminopterin, to treat children with acute lymphatic leukemia. In many of the subsequent studies over the next decade, single agents were used to induce a remission and therapy was then stopped until there was recurrence of the disease (Table I). The most effective single agents were prednisone and vincristine which induced remission in 60% to 70% of the children.

Table I

REMISSION INDUCTION: SINGLE AGENTS
SELECTED EXAMPLES

Drug	Dosage	Regimen	Complete Remission (%)	Selected References
Prednisone	60 mg/m^2	4 ÷ dose/day po	70	2-5
Vincristine	1.5 mg/m^2	Weekly IV	60	6-9
L-Asparaginase	10,000 U/m^2	2-3 X's/week IM	60	10,11
Cyclophosphamide	150 mg/m^2	Daily	40	12-14
Daunorubicin	50 mg/m^2	Daily X's 3,4	30	15-17
Doxorubicin	30 mg/m^2	Daily X's 3,4	30	18-20
6-Mercaptopurine	75 mg/m^2	Daily	30	21-23
Methotrexate	3 mg/m^2	Daily	30	22,24
Arabinosyl Cytosine	100 mg/m^2	Daily X's 5	20	25-27

2. MAINTENANCE THERAPY - MULTIAGENT

The use of a combination of agents is much more effective (Table II); vincristine and prednisone together induce remission in 85% of the children and vincristine, prednisone with L-asparaginase or daunomycin induces remission in about 90%. Clinically there is a fantastic response to these agents with rapid disappearance of blasts from the peripheral blood, resolution of organomegaly and return to normal marrow morphology function within four weeks. The leukemia cell burden has been reduced by at least 95%, that is, from about a 1 kg leukemic mass to a 50 gm leukemic mass or less. From the cancer biologist's point of view, adapting Skipper's mouse model (48) to a child model, the leukemia cell burden has only been reduced from 10^{12} cells to less than $5x10^{10}$ cells or at least "1-1/2 logs" with "10-1/2 logs" to go.

Table II

REMISSION INDUCTION - MULTI AGENT
SELECTED EXAMPLES

Agents	Complete Remission (%)	References
Prednisone + Cyclophosphamide	75	28,29
Prednisone + 6-Mercaptopurine	80	28-32
Prednisone + Methotrexate	80	29,31
Prednisone + Vincristine	85	33-35
Prednisone + Daunorubicin	85	36,37
Prednisone + Vincristine + Daunomycin	91	38-40
Prednisone + Vincristine + L-Asparaginase	93	41-43
Prednisone + Vincristine + L-Asparaginase + Daunorubicin	95	44,45
Vincristine + Cyclophosphamide	52	46
6-Mercaptopurine + Methotrexate	43	47

3. MAINTENANCE THERAPY - SINGLE AGENTS

The next major advance that was made was the use of maintenance therapy to sustain remission. In studies by both Freireich et al. (2) and the investigators at the Southwest Oncology Group (29), it was shown that the duration of remission was longer in those children randomized to continuous 6-mercaptopurine chemotherapy as compared to the children receiving no maintenance therapy, two months of maintenance chemotherapy, or six months of maintenance chemotherapy. The duration of remission in children receiving a single maintenance agent therapy is given in Table III. Goldin and colleagues (53) reported that methotrexate was more effective when given on an intermittent schedule than a daily oral schedule in studies in mice with early disease. In a comparison of an intermittent schedule and a daily oral schedule the Cancer and Leukemia Group B investigators (49) obtained a median duration of remission

Table III

REMISSION MAINTENANCE: SINGLE AGENTS
SELECTED EXAMPLES

Agent	Schedule	MDR* (Months)	References
None	---	2-3	2-4
Prednisone	Daily, oral	2	3,5
Cyclophosphamide	Daily, oral	3	28
6-Mercaptopurine	Daily, oral	5	2,22,28
Methotrexate	Daily, oral	3	22,49
Methotrexate	2 X/week	10	49
Methotrexate	Every 2 weeks	11	39,50
Methotrexate	5 day course every 2 weeks	10	51
Vincristine	Weekly	10	52

* MDR - median duration of remission

of eleven months and two months, respectively. Subsequently, reports of further success with combination chemotherapy used during maintenance began to appear.

4. MUTANT CLONES

At this point it would be helpful to again consider the mouse/child model as to why combination chemotherapy should be more effective. As mentioned before, the child has around 10^{12} cells at the time of diagnosis. In animal and *in vitro* studies, a mutational event may occur in every 10^5 or 10^6 cells (54). In Figure 1 the exponential proliferation that may occur in a child with acute leukemia is shown with the mutational events developing during the course of the leukemic cell proliferation.

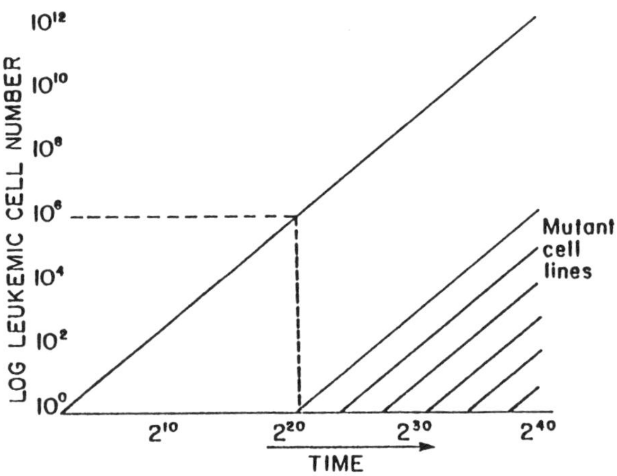

Figure 1. Mutational events that occur during the exponential growth of leukemic cells in a child who has 10^{12} leukemic cells at diagnosis.

When remission is induced with prednisone alone approximately 60% of the children will achieve remission, but within two months half will have relapsed even if prednisone is continued (3). If, on the other hand, predisone and 6-mercaptopurine are used to induce remission and the remission is maintained with 6-mercaptopurine and methotrexate, the median duration of remission is 11 months and 5% or more of the children will be cured of their disease (32). Figure 2 is a diagrammatic representation of the reduction of malignant cells that has occurred using vincristine and prednisone for remission induction, and 6-mercaptopurine for maintenance therapy. In this example 10^7 cells of a mutant clone resistant to 6-mercaptopurine was present at diagnosis. This resulted in recurrence of clinical evidence of disease at 28 weeks; otherwise all malignant cells would have been eliminated by 32 weeks.

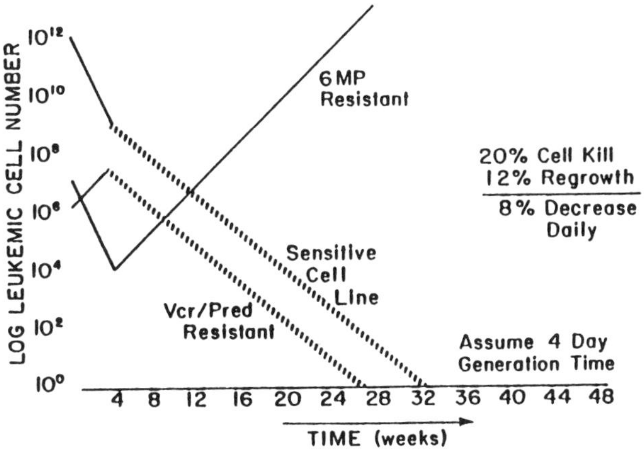

Figure 2. Diagramatic representation of the reduction of leukemic cells in a child with 10^{12} leukemic cells at diagnosis. Remission is induced with vincristine (Vcr) and prednisone (Pred) in the first 4 weeks. Maintenance therapy with daily oral 6-mercaptopurine (6MP) reduces the 6MP sensitive cell lines to one cell by 32 weeks. Unfortunately, a mutant clone resistant to 6MP results in recurrence of disease.

5. KINETICS OF CELL KILL

Figure 3 attempts to examine in more detail the reduction of leukemic cells that occurs with daily therapy. The generation time for leukemic cells as reported by Mauer, et al. (55,56) and others (57-61), is probably around 60-70 hours and the time during DNA synthesis is about 20 hours. In Figure 3 it is assumed that the DNA synthesis time was 20 hours, but there was cell progression delay due to a block at the G1-S junction due to the therapeutic agent used and the resulting generation time was 96 hours. The results shown are those that would result in a 30%, 20% and 15% cell kill with an agent given daily over a six hour period if the generation time is four days. In the first example, the child would be cured of his disease in approximately 150 days if 10^{12} cells were present at diagnosis. In the example of a 15% cell kill daily, which might occur if only 50% of the cells were proliferating, there would be a 3% daily decrease in leukemic cells. It would take over 900 days to reduce the leukemic cell population to 0 providing the non-proliferative cells were gradually recruited and began to proliferate during the course of therapy.

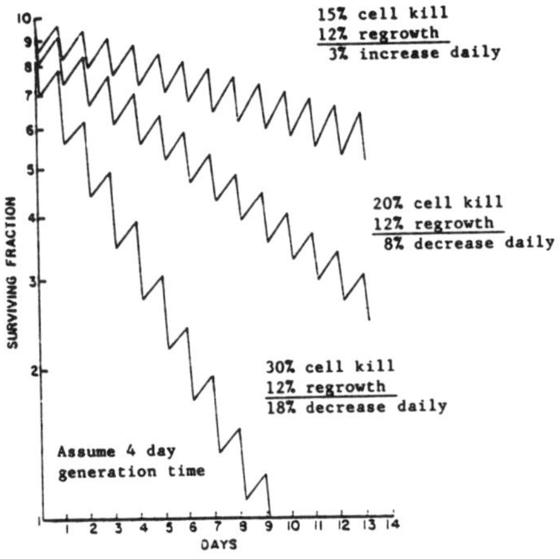

Figure 3. Reduction of leukemic cells in a host treated with a cytocidal "S-phase" specific agent for six hours daily.

The equations used to estimate the length of time to cure or to relapse are derived as follows. Let T_O be the cell generation time, and L_O the length of time lethal drug levels are maintained. All time is assumed to be in hours, treatment is administered every 24 hours and $L_O < 24$. Let C_O be the number of leukemic cells present at initiation of treatment and C_n, $n \geq 1$, be the number of leukemic cells present at the end of the nth day (treatment). Let K be the proportion of cells going through DNA synthesis (or sensitive to the cytocidal agent). From the following it is noted that each day $(24-L_O)/T_O$ of cells not killed by the treatment will divide before the next drug dose is administered.

```
<------------ To------------>
<-- Lo -->
<------- 24 hrs ------->
<- - - - - - - - - - - - - - - - - - ->
                Time
```

Thus, at the end of day 1, there will be

$$C_1 = ((1-K)C_O + (24-L_O)/T_O)(1-K)C_O$$

surviving leukemic cells. The first term on the right hand side of the equation is the number of cells surviving the therapy and the second term is the number of cells produced by cell division which occurred after therapy was stopped and before the next dose was administered. Since C_O was the number of leukemic cells at the beginning of day 1 and K, L_O and T_O are fixed from day to day, we get the following general equation:

$$C_n = [(1-K)\ [1 + (24-L_O)T_O]]^n C_O, \quad n \geq 1$$

To derive results of the first example, let $T_O = 96$ hours, $L_O = 6$ hours, $K = 0.3$ (30% cell kill) and $C_O = 10^{12}$ cells.

Then

$$C_n = [0.7(1.1875)]^n \times 10^{12}$$

To find how many days are required to eradicate all but the last leukemic cell, we set $C_n = 1$ and solve for n. Hence

$$[.8313]^n \times 10^{12} = 1; \quad n = 150 \text{ days}$$

or 150 days are required to reduce the number of leukemic cells to one.

At the time of diagnosis of leukemia, less than 5-15% of the malignant cells are proliferating, although this is frequently higher at the time of relapse (55-60). Some investigators feel that a large non-proliferating pool remains even when the cell numbers have been reduced to below 10^{10} cells. In the studies done by Edelstein, Valeriote and Vietti (62) a significant non-proliferative fraction of L1210 could not be detected after prolonged infusions of cytosine arabinoside in mice with advance disease until the cell population had been reduced by four or five "logs" (Fig. 4).

The differences between the theoretical curves and actual curves for both mouse and human leukemia were discussed by Skipper, Schabel, et al. (48,64-66). They noted that the theoretical curve of the percent of unlabelled cells was significantly different from the actual curve after continuous _in vivo_ exposure of leukemic cells to tritiated thymidine (Fig. 5). Similarly the theoretical curve for the effect of an every three hour exposure of L1210 cells to Ara-C was very different than the observed curves obtained from both _in vivo_ and _in vitro_ studies (Fig. 6). These studies indicate that in order to maximize cell kill, the exposure to a phase specific agent must be for a much longer time than the estimated generation time.

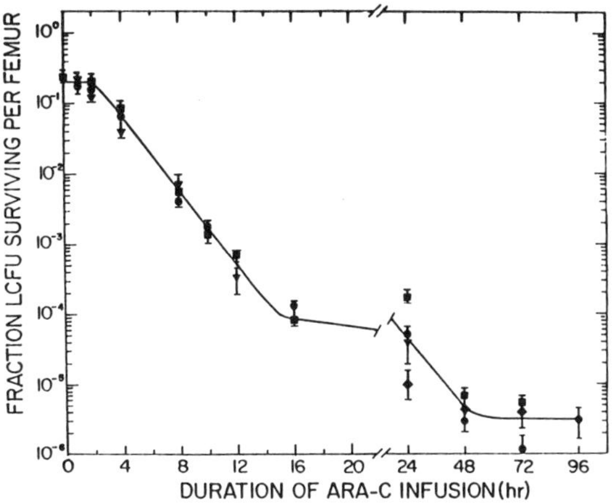

Figure 4. Surviving fraction of leukemia colony forming units (LCFU) as a function of duration of infusion of 2 mg arabinosyl cytosine (ARA-C) per mouse. Different symbols represent different experiments: errors are ± 1 S.E. From Ref. 63.

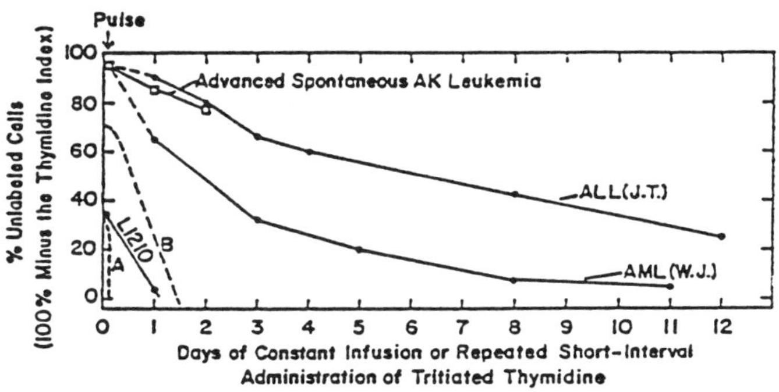

Figure 5. Fractional survival curves of L1210 leukemic cell populations observed on exposure to maximally effective concentrations of arabinosyl cytosine; and theoretical survival curves calculated on a no-range basis. NOTE: One might anticipate an even greater deviation for acute lymphocytic leukemia or acute myelocytic leukemia populations than is observed for L1210 leukemia. It is assumed that the survival curves for L1210 leukemic cells constantly exposed to arabinosyl cytosine are a reflection of a) the leukemic cells in S-phase at the start of exposure, and b) 1.0 minus the cumulative distribution of TG_1 + TM + TG_2 in the remaining viable cells. From Ref. 67.

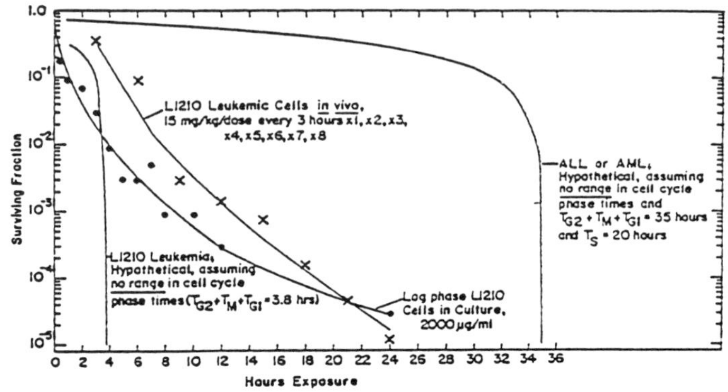

Figure 6. Decrease in unlabeled cells of L1210, advanced spontaneous AK, and advanced human acute leukemias on constant exposure to tritiated thymidine versus hypothetical decreases calculated on a no-range basis. A. Hypothetical decrease in unlabeled cells with time calculated on a no-range basis for L1210 leukemia. B. Hypothetical decrease in unlabeled cells with time calculated on a no-range basis for acute lymphocytic leukemia or acute myelocytic leukemia. From Ref. 67.

6. MAINTENANCE THERAPY - MULTIAGENT

Dr. Zeulzer and colleagues at the Children's Hospital of Michigan (32) were among the first investigators to use multiple drugs to maintain a remission. They induced remission with 6-mercaptopurine and prednisone and then subsequently maintained the remission with sequential 3 month cycles of daily oral 6-mercaptopurine and daily oral methotrexate. The median duration of remission for these children was 11 months. Freireich and colleagues at the NCI (68) gave an intensive intermittent cyclic combination of four agents (VAMP - vincristine, amethopterin, 6-mercaptopurine and prednisone) for six months to children with acute lymphatic leukemia and obtained a median remission of ten months. From these studies they observed the median time to relapse occurred about four months after cessation of therapy. Assuming a 96 hour doubling time, they theorized that VAMP had reduced the leukemic population to less than 10 cells. The NCI investigators (69) then devised a new regimen with the same agents (POMP - Purinethol, Oncovin, methotrexate and prednisone) and administered the combination for 14 months. The median duration of remission for these patients was 13-1/2 months.

Other combinations of therapy for maintenance, the addition of intensive consolidation therapy, combinations of cyclic therapy and superimposition of other agents on single or multi-agent therapy did not convincingly prolong the subsequent remission and the number of long term survivors in these studies remained disappointingly low (70).

7. CENTRAL NERVOUS SYSTEM DISEASE

With this increase in the median duration of remission from four to six months to over a year, the incidence of CNS disease markedly increased (71). Figures 7 and 8 are an attempt to show why this might occur. In a patient with good prognosis (Fig. 7), replication occurs primarily in the bone marrow. The cells leave the bone marrow and spread to the intravascular spaces, lymph nodes and lymphatics just as the normal precursors would do. Minimal proliferation probably occurs in these locations. The leukemic cells, just as for their normal counterparts, also pass into pharmacologic sanctuaries, the principle of which is the central nervous system. Although we know that about 5% of the children have overt CNS disease at diagnosis, active proliferation in these areas is less than in the bone marrow (26,72). With time, these malignant cells, if left untreated in the pharmacologic sanctuaries, will cause CNS relapse, testicular relapse, or possibly, if a mutational event occurs, a resistant strain might pass back into the peripheral blood and into the bone marrow despite continued therapy where they will cause recurrence of marrow disease. Figure 8 is that of a patient with poor prognosis. Not only is there increased proliferation in the bone marrow but proliferation is also accelerated in the blood, lymphatics and lymph nodes and there are an increased number of cells which pass into the pharmacologic sanctuaries.

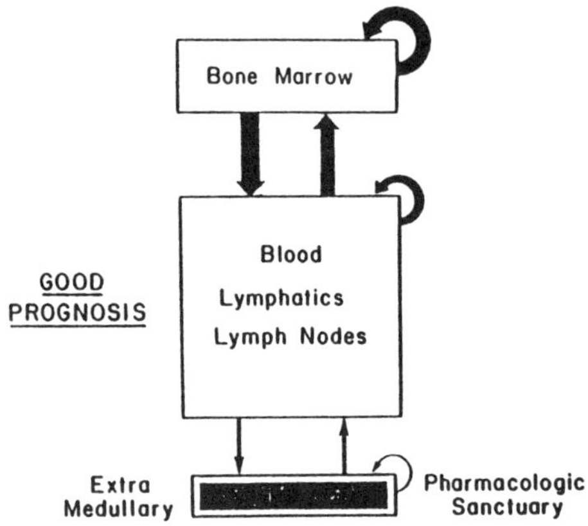

Figure 7. "Good" prognosis - acute lymphatic leukemia. This diagram is drawn to suggest that proliferation of blast cells is primarily occurring in the bone marrow. Malignant cells diffuse freely into the vascular lymphatic systems and there is some diffusion into the extramedullary areas. Replicating is primarily limited to the bone marrow, although some does occur in other areas.

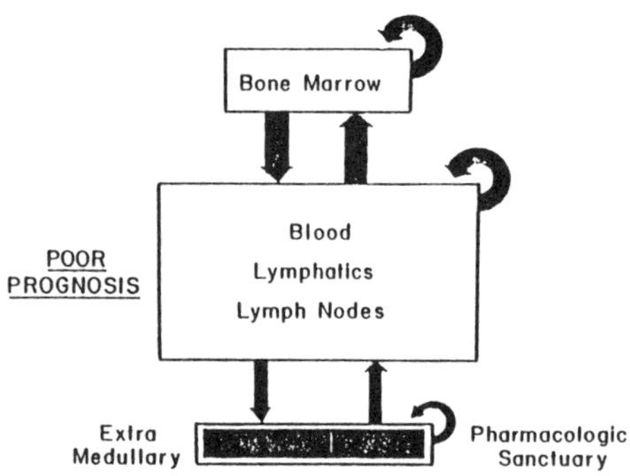

Figure 8. "Poor" prognosis - acute lymphatic leukemia. The number of malignant cells in the bone marrow compartment of a child with poor prognosis is the same as in the child with good prognosis, but the number of cells circulating in the blood, lymphatics and lymph nodes is much greater. Similarly, there is a much greater diffusion into the pharmacologic sanctuaries. Replication occurs at an increased rate both in the systemic circulation and the extramedullary areas.

8. CONTROL OF CENTRAL NERVOUS SYSTEM DISEASE

The animal model for the management of occult central nervous system disease was proposed by Johnson (74). He treated mice with advanced L1210 disease of the central nervous system with radiation and combination chemotherapy and effected a significant number of cures. Using the ideas behind this model Dr. Pinkel and his colleagues at St. Jude (35,41,63,67,75-78) made the next and one of the most significant advances in the treatment of children with acute lymphatic leukemia. Through a series of studies they showed that cranial spinal irradiation or cranial irradiation and a course of intrathecal methotrexate therapy added to multi-agent induction therapy and to multi-agent maintenance therapy, not only controlled CNS disease and markedly prolonged the median duration of remission, but also significantly increased the number of cures. The results from some of their most significant studies are shown in Table IV. From their studies, vincristine, prednisone and L-asparaginase with cranial irradiation, 2400 rad, and a course of intrathecal methotrexate followed by maintenance therapy with 6-mercaptopurine daily and methotrexate weekly will result in a survival rate of over 50% of the children with acute leukemia. The addition of an intensive consolidation regimen or the addition of other agents to the 6-mercaptopurine/methotrexate maintenance regimen did not improve the results.

Another very effective regimen was developed by the investigators at Sloan-Kettering (79-82). This regimen (termed the LSA_2L_2 regimen), used vincristine, prednisone, cyclophosphamide and daunomycin to induce remission, arabinosyl cytosine, 6-thioguanine, L-asparaginase and BCNU to consolidate the induction followed by a multi-agent remission maintenance therapy. Intrathecal methotrexate was given during induction, consolidation and maintenance. More than 50% of the children entered on this protocol remained in continuous complete remission over five years.

Table IV

"TOTAL THERAPY" STUDIES BY ST. JUDE CHILDREN'S HOSPITAL*

Study	Induction	Consolidation Phase	CNS Therapy	Maintenance Therapy	Reinforcement Therapy	Comments
V	P + V	IV 6-MP/d x 3 IV MTX/d x 3 IV CYC/d x 1	Skull 2400 R + I.T. MTX	PO 6-MP/day IV MTX/week IV CYC/week	P + V 2 wks every 10 wks	54% CR >5 yrs
VI	P + V + D	None - Or - IV 6-MP/d x 3 IV MTX/d x 3 IV CYC/d x 1	None - Or - 2400 R Craniospinal	PO 6-MP/day PO MTX/week PO CYC/week	P + V 2 wks every 10 wks	No CNS therapy - 9/46 in cont. CR CNS therapy - MDR is >5 yrs
VII	P + V	None	2400 R Craniospinal - Or - 2400 R skull + I.T. MTX	PO 6-MP/day PO MTX/week PO CYC/week	None - Or - P + V 2 wks every 10 wks	41/94 in CR for 21+ - 39+ mo No difference
VIII	P + V + L-Asp	None	2400 R skull + I.T. MTX	1-IV MTX/week 2-PO 6-MP/d +1 3-IV CYC/wk +2 4-IV Ara-C/wk +3	None	1-MDR = 12 mo 2-MDR >5 yrs 3-MDR = 35 mo 4-MDR = 38 mo

Abbreviations:
CNS = central nervous system
P = prednisone
V = vincristine
D = daunomycin
R = rad
6-MP = 6-mercaptopurine
MTX = methotrexate
CYC = cyclophosphamide
L-Asp = L-Asparaginase
Ara-C = arabinosylcytosine
CR = complete remission
MDR = median duration of remission

* References 41, 63, 76

The pediatric investigators in Acute Leukemia Group B (42) and the Southwest Oncology Group (83) (now both of the Pediatric Oncology Group), developed effective systemic maintenance regimens with maintenance intrathecal methotrexate. Generally, a course of intrathecal methotrexate consisting of five or six weekly doses is given when the remission is obtained and followed by periodic intrathecal methotrexate along with systemic maintenance therapy. The most effective to date is the regimen (Fig. 9) initially piloted by Dr. Sullivan and colleagues at M.D. Anderson and later adopted by the Pediatric Oncology Group as one of their standard regimens (83). The patients receiving this regimen are induced into remission with vincristine and prednisone, consolidated with cyclophosphamide and L-asparaginase followed by triple agent intrathecal therapy and intensive IV methotrexate, and then maintained on 6-mercaptopurine daily, weekly methotrexate, periodic prednisone reinforcement and triple agent intrathecal maintenance therapy.

INDUCTION:	V + P	
CONSOLIDATION:	L-Asp DAILY x 14 CYC DAYS 1 AND 14 ↓	
	TIT DAY 1 MTX DAYS 2, 3, 4, AND 5	EVERY TWO WEEKS
MAINTENANCE:	6MP DAILY MTX WEEKLY TIT EVERY 8 WEEKS	
REINFORCEMENT:	PREDNISONE DAILY FOR 4 WEEKS	EVERY 16 WEEKS

Figure 9. This regimen developed by Sullivan et al. at M.D. Anderson Hospital is a very effective antileukemic regimen which uses triple drug intrathecal therapy initially during consolidation and then every 8 weeks during 3 years of maintenance therapy.

Abbreviations: V = vincristine; P = prednisone; L-Asp = L-Asparaginase; CYC = cyclophosphamide; TIT = triple intrathecal therapy; MTX = methotrexate; 6MP = 6-mercaptopurine

Freeman and his colleagues (84) at Roswell Park developed a prophylactic CNS regimen using intermediate dose methotrexate with intrathecal therapy every two weeks for three courses as a consolidation followed by 6-mercaptopurine daily and methotrexate weekly maintenance. The Cancer and Leukemia Group B investigators (85) compared this regimen to a similar regimen except that one-half of the patients received cranial irradiation therapy and intrathecal methotrexate as CNS prophylaxis. The median duration of remission for both groups is similar, but the incidence of CNS relapse was much higher for the group receiving the intermediate dose methotrexate + intrathecal methotrexate, whereas the incidence of bone marrow relapse and testicular relapse is higher for the children receiving cranial irradiation and a course of intrathecal methotrexate. Subsequently, a study at Roswell Park Memorial Institute (86) comparing six courses of intermediate dose methotrexate/intrathecal methotrexate with three courses of intermediate dose methotrexate/intrathecal methotrexate revealed a significant improvement in the relapse free survival (Fig. 10).

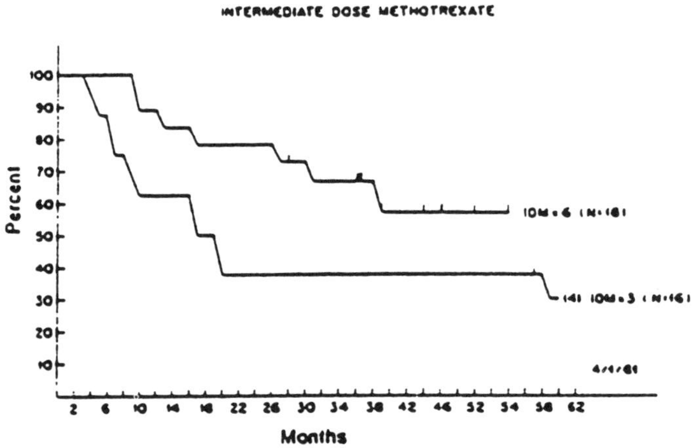

Figure 10. Disease free survival in patients treated with 3 or 6 courses of intermediate dose methotrexate (IDM) from Green et al.

Children's Cancer Study Group investigators observed that a short course of intrathecal methotrexate without maintenance intrathecal therapy was markedly inadequate therapy for children with WBC $\geq$ 20,000/ul when compared to cranial irradiation and intrathecal methotrexate or cranial spinal irradiation therapy (87) (Fig. 11). They demonstrated in a subsequent study that 1800 rad cranial irradiation plus intrathecal methotrexate is just as effective as 2400 rad plus intrathecal methotrexate and many studies now use this lower radiation therapy dose (88).

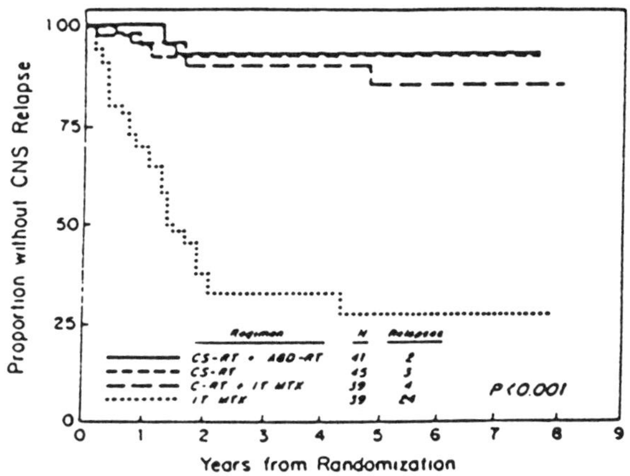

Figure 11. Time to isolated CNS relapse in children with an initial WBC $\geq$ 20,000/ul (from Ref. 87).
CS = RT + ABD RT = craniospinal radiation therapy + abdominal radiation therapy
CS = RT = craniospinal radiation therapy
C - RT + IT MTX = cranial radiation therapy + intrathecal methotrexate
IT MTX = intrathecal methotrexate

9. RECENT PROGRESS

Dr. Sallan and colleagues (89) at Boston reported an interesting study. Children were induced into remission with vincristine, prednisone and doxorubicin. During consolidation, all received L-asparaginase and cranial irradiation plus a course of intrathecal methotrexate for central nervous system prophylaxis. All were then given a six month intensification course with vincristine, prednisone and doxorubicin; one half also received L-aspariginase. Maintenance therapy for all consisted of intermittent courses of 6-mercaptopurine, methotrexate, prednisone and vincristine (Fig. 12). The disease free survival for the children receiving L-asparaginase during their intensification regimen was significantly longer than the other group (Fig.

13). Figures 14 and 15 are an attempt to explain these results by using the mouse/child model. Neither vincristine, prednisone, nor doxorubicin are thought to be good remission maintenance agents, although individually and especially in combination they are effective remission induction agents. This failure to maintain remission is apparently due to the fact that a significant number of leukemic cells have mutated to strains that are resistant to these agents. L-asparaginase is also probably an ineffective remission maintenance agent but the leukemic cells, resistant to vincristine + prednisone + doxorubicin, presumably are not resistant to L-asparaginase, or at least they do not proliferate in the presence of L-asparaginase.

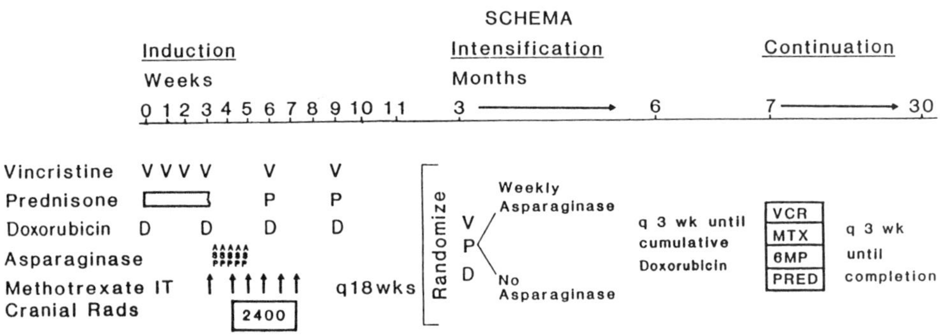

Figure 12. Chemotherapy schema used by investigators at Boston in ramdomized trial to assess the therapeutic efficacy of weekly L-asparaginase added to an intensification regimen (VPDA) compared to a control arm (VPD). From Ref. 89.

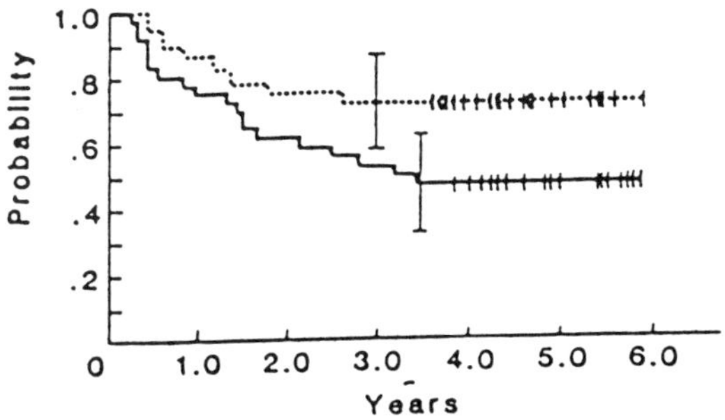

RX	CCR	Fail	Total
—— VPD	17	19	36
...... VPDA	26	10	36

7/83

Figure 13. Disease free survival in children treated with VPDA compared to group receiving VPD (see Fig. 12) (P = 0.04). From Ref. 89.

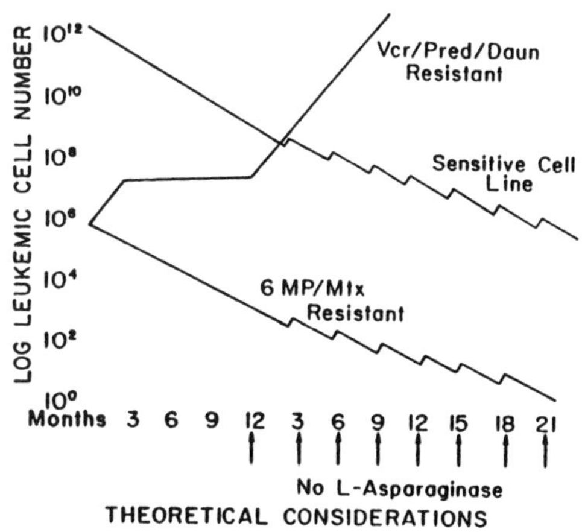

Figure 14. Theoretical reduction in leukemic cell population which occurred after remission induction and consolidation with a regimen proposed by Sallan and colleagues at Boston (89). This theoretical child had recurrence of disease after 9 weeks of therapy because of mutant strain resistant to vincristine, prednisone and daunomycin.

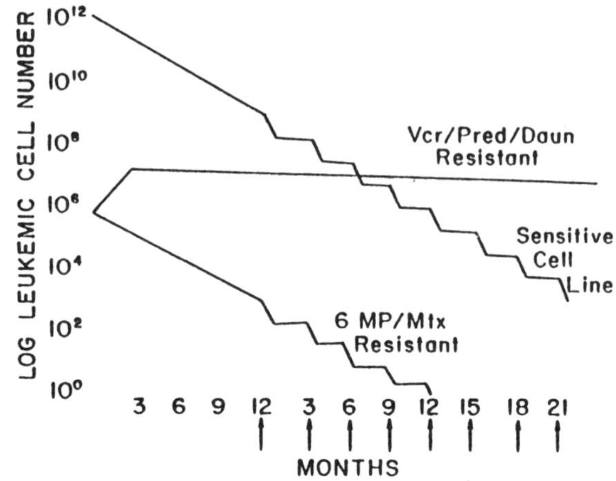

Figure 15. This child was treated with the same regimen except that L-asparaginase was added to the intensification phase and controlled the proliferation of the vincristine, prednisone, daunomycin resistant strain.

The Berlin-Frankfort-Munich (BFM) investigators (44,45) have reported on their intensive remission and intensive consolidation regimens. Patients are induced into remission with prednisone, vincristine, daunomycin and L-asparaginase for four weeks followed by cyclophosphamide, arabinosyl cytosine, 6-mercaptopurine, intrathecal methotrexate and cranial irradiation for four weeks. After achieving remission those with poor prognosis received an intensive consolidation therapy consisting of dexamethasone, vincristine, doxorubicin and L-asparaginase for four weeks followed by cyclophosphamide, arabinosyl cytosine, intrathecal methotrexate and 6-thioguanine for an additional two weeks. All patients were then maintained on 6-mercaptopurine daily orally and methotrexate weekly for two and a half years. All patients also received three courses of prednisone and vincristine reinforcement during the first year. Over 75% of the patients, including good and poor prognosis, entered on these studies are still in continuous complete remission.

The principal cause of failure remains the recurrence of the disease due to development of resistant mutant clones. The use of a multiagent intensive consolidation, as in the BFM studies, may irradicate mutant clones. Not only is there a search for new agents which might be (more) effective but also, standard agents are being reevaluated to determine if their therapeutic efficacy can be improved. Examples are high dose methotrexate with L-asparaginase rescue (90), the combination of methotrexate and arabinosyl cytosine (91), arabinosyl cytosine plus L-asparaginase (92), and prolonged infusions of 6-mercaptopurine (93).

10. THOUGHTS FOR FUTURE STUDIES

In patients with poor prognosis who relapse in the first six months, the possibility of an unusually short generation time rather than drug resistance should be considered. As an example, an effective phase specific oral agent would fail to control the leukemic cell population if the generation time was 36 hours, the DNA synthesis time 10 hours, and lethal levels were achieved for only a four hour time interval. Thus, if in the general equation, we let T_O = 36 hours, L_O = 4 hours, K = (10/36) = .28 and $C_O = 5x10^{10}$ cells, the number of leukemic cells at the end of n days would be

$$C_n = [.72(1.5556)]^n \, 5x10^{10} = [1.12]^n \times 5x10^{10}$$

Since there is a net cell increase each day, n would be the number of days until the tumor burden is 10^{12} cells, i.e., relapse. Hence,

$$[1.12]^n \times 5x10^{10} = 10^{12}; \quad n = 27 \text{ days}$$

The child would be in frank relapse in approximately 27 days. In these patients, agents should probably be administered as prolonged three or four day infusions.

Although the incidence of central nervous system relapse has decreased from the highs of 40 to 60% to less than 10%, there is still some concern that the pharmacologic sanctuaries may serve as a reservoir. Mutant strains could develop in these sanctuaries with subsequent marrow relapse when they returned to the systemic circulation and to the bone marrow. The study by Willoughby and colleagues for the Medical Research Council (94) suggests a clue for future studies. In this study, patients who developed overt CNS leukemia were induced into remission with intrathecal methotrexate and then randomized to receive cranial irradiation or craniospinal irradiation. The incidence of CNS relapse as a first event was low in both groups but the duration of the subsequent bone marrow remission was much longer in the patients who received craniospinal radiation. This suggests that tissues lying along the spinal axis may act as pharmacologic sanctuaries for leukemic cells.

11. SUMMARY

In the past and still today, most of the therapeutic regimens have been developed on an empiric basis. We should go back to the child/mouse model and try to develop plausible reasons as to why we fail as well as why we suceed. This will enable us to devise therapeutic regimens to test specific hypotheses and will lead to the development of more effective therapy.

ACKNOWLEDGEMENT

This has been partially supported by NCI grants CA-30969, CA-05587 and CA-29139.

REFERENCES

1. Farber S, Diamond et al: Temporary remissions in acute leukemia in children produced by folic acid antagonist, 4-amino-pteroyl-glutamic acid (aminopterin). N. Eng. J. Med. 238:787-793, 1948.
2. Freireich EJ, Gehan E, Frei E III et al: The effect of 6-mercaptopurine on the duration of steroid-induced remission in acute leukemia: A model for evaluation of other potentially useful therapy. Blood 21:699-716, 1963.
3. Hyman CB, Borda E et al: Prednisone in childhood leukemia; comparison of interrupted and continuous therapy. Pediatrics 24:1005-1008, 1959.
4. Vietti TJ, Sullivan MP, Berry DH et al: The response of acute childhood leukemia to an initial and a second course of prednisone. J. Pediatr. 66:18-26, 1965.
5. Wolff JA, Brubaker CA, Murphy ML et al: Prednisone therapy of acute childhood leukemia: Prognosis and duration of response in 330 treated patients. J. Pediatr. 70:626-631, 1967.
6. Evans AE, Farber S, Brunet S, Mariano PJ: Vincristine in the treatment of acute leukemia in children. Cancer 16: 1302-1306, 1963.
7. Haggard ME, Fernbach DJ, Holcomb TM et al: Vincristine in acute leukemia of childhood. Cancer 22:438-444, 1968.
8. Heyn RM, Beatty EC Jr, Hammond D et al: Vincristine in the treatment of acute leukemia. Pediatrics 38:82-91, 1966.
9. Karon M, Freireich EJ, Frei E III et al: The role of vincristine in the treatment of childhood acute leukemia. Clin. Pharmacol. Ther. 7:332-339, 1966.
10. Ertel IJ, Nesbit MG, Hammond D et al: Effective dose of L-asparaginase for induction of remission in previously treated children with acute leukemia: A report from Children's Cancer Study Group. Cancer Res. 39:3893-3896, 1979.
11. Sutow WW, Garcia F, Starling KA et al: L-asparaginase therapy in children with advanced leukemia. Cancer 28: 819-824, 1971.
12. Fernbach DJ, Sutow WW, Thurman WG, Vietti TJ: Clinical evaluation of cyclophosphamide, a new agent for the treatment of children with acute leukemia. JAMA 182:30-37, 1962.
13. Holcomb TM: Cyclophosphamide (NSC-26271) in the treatment of acute leukemia in children. Cancer Chemother. Rep. 51: 389-392, 1967.
14. Pierce MI, Shore N, Sitarz A et al: Cyclophosphamide therapy in acute leukemia of childhood. Cancer 19:1551-1560, 1966.
15. Holton CP, Lonsdale D, Nora AH et al: Clinical study of daunomycin (NSC-82151) in children with acute leukemia. Cancer 22:1014-1017, 1968.

16. Jones B, Holland JF, Morrison AR: Daunomycin in the treatment of resistant acute lymphoblastic leukemia. Cancer Res. 31:84-90, 1971.
17. Tan C, Tasaka H, Yu KP et al: Daunomycin, an antitumor antibiotic, in the treatment of neoplastic disease. Cancer 20:333-353, 1967.
18. Ragab AH, Sutow WW, Komp DM, Starling KA, Lyon GM, George S: Adriamycin in the treatment of childhood acute leukemia. Cancer 36:1123-1126, 1975.
19. Starling KA, Berry DH, Britton HA, Humphrey GB, Vats T, Ragab AH: Three dose regimens of adriamycin for induction of remission in acute leukemia in children. Med. Pediatr. Onc. 1:271-276, 1975.
20. Tan C, Rosen G, Charini F, Haghbin M, Helson L, Wollner N, Murphy ML: Adriamycin (NSC-123127) in pediatric malignancies. Cancer Chemother. Rep. 6:259-266, 1975.
21. Boggs D, Wintrobe MW, Cartwright GE: The acute leukemias. Medicine 41:163-225, 1962.
22. Frei E III, Freireich EJ, Gehan E et al: (Acute Leukemia Cooperative Group B): Studies of sequential and combination antimetabolite therapy in acute leukemia: 6-mercaptopurine and methotrexate, from the Acute Leukemia Group B. Blood 18:431-454, 1961.
23. Sullivan MP, Beatty EC Jr, Hyman CB et al: A comparison of the effectiveness of standard dose 6-mercaptopurine, combination 6-mercaptopurine and DON, and high-loading 6-mercaptopurine therapies in treatment of the acute leukemias of childhood: Results of a cooperative study. Cancer Chemother. Rep. 18:83-95, 1962.
24. Holland JF: Symposium on the experimental pharmacology and clinical use of antimetabolites. VIII. Folic acid antagonists. Clin. Pharmacol. Ther. 2:374-409, 1961.
25. Howard JP, Albo V, Newton WA Jr: Cytosine arabinoside results of a cooperative study in acute childhood leukemia. Cancer 21:341-345, 1968.
26. Traggis DG, Dohlwitz A, Das L, Jaffe N, Moloney WC, Hall TC: Cytosine arabinoside in acute leukemia of childhood. Cancer 28:815-818, 1971.
27. Wang JJ, Selawry OS, Bodey GP, Vietti TJ: Prolonged infusion of arabinosyl cytosine in childhood leukemia. Cancer 25:1-6, 1970.
28. Fernbach DJ, Griffith KM, Haggard ME et al: Chemotherapy of acute leukemia in childhood: Comparison of cyclophosphamide and mercaptopurine. N. Eng. J. Med. 275:451-456, 1966.
29. Lonsdale D, Gehan EA, Fernbach DJ et al: Interrupted vs. continued maintenance therapy in childhood acute leukemia. Cancer 36:341-352, 1975.
30. Fernbach DJ, George SL, Sutow WW et al: Long-term results of reinforcement therapy in children with acute leukemia. Cancer 36:1552-1559, 1975.

31. Krivit W, Brubaker C, Thatcher LG et al: Maintenance therapy in acute leukemia of children. Comparison of cyclic vs. sequential methods. Cancer 21:352-356, 1968.
32. Zuelzer WW: Implications of long-term survival in acute leukemia of childhood treated with composite cyclic therapy. Blood 24:477-494, 1964.
33. Berry DH, Pullen J, George S, Vietti TJ, Sullivan MP, Fernbach D: Comparison of prednisone, vincristine, methotrexate and 6-mercaptopurine versus vincristine and prednisone induction therapy in childhood acute leukemia. Cancer 36:98-102, 1975.
34. Komp DM, George SL, Falletta JM et al: Cyclophosphamide-asparaginase-vincristine-prednisone induction therapy in childhood acute lymphocytic and non-lymphocytic leukemia. Cancer 37:1243-1247, 1976.
35. Pinkel D: The treatment of childhood acute lymphocytic leukemia. In: Modern Trends in Human Leukemia III, Neth R, Gallo RC, Hofschneider P-H et al (eds), Berlin, Springer-Verlag, 1979, p.81.
36. Holton CP, Vietti TJ, Nora AH et al: Daunomycin and prednisone for induction of remission in advanced leukemia. N. Engl. J. Med. 280:171-174, 1969.
37. Sackman-Muriel F, Svarch E, Helft ME et al: Evaluation of intensification and maintenance programs in the treatment of acute lymphoblastic leukemia. Cancer 42:1730-1740, 1978.
38. Jacquillat C, Weil M, Gemon MF et al: Combination therapy in 130 patients with acute lymphoblastic leukemia (Protocol 06 LA 66-Paris). Cancer Res. 33:3278-3284, 1973.
39. Pavlovsky S, Penalver J, Epping-Helft M et al: Induction and maintenance of remission in acute leukemia. Effectiveness of combination therapy in 227 cases. Cancer 31:273-279, 1973.
40. Vietti TJ, Starling K, Wilber K, Lonsdale D, Lane DM: Vincristine, prednisone and daunomycin in acute leukemia of childhood. Cancer 27:602-607, 1971.
41. Aur RJA, Simone JV, Verzosa MS et al: Childhood acute lymphocytic leukemia: Study VIII. Cancer 42:2123, 1978.
42. Jones B, Holland JF, Jacquillat C et al: Optimal use of L-asparaginase (NSC-109229) in acute lymphocytic leukemia. Med. Pediatr. Oncol. 3:387-400, 1977.
43. Ortega JA, Nesbit ME Jr, Donaldson MH et al: L-asparaginase, vincristine and prednisone for induction of first remission in acute lymphocytic leukemia. Cancer Res. 37:535-540, 1977.
44. Henze G, Langermann et al: Evgebuisse der studie BFM 76/79 zur behandlung der akutsu lymphoblastischen leukamie bei kindern und jugendlochen. Klin. Padiatr. 193:145-154, 1981.

45. Riehm H, Gadner H et al: Acute lymphoblastic leukemia: Treatment results in three BFM studies (1970-1981). In: Leukemia Research: Advances in Cell Biology and Treatment, Murphy S, Gilbert JR (eds), Elsevier Science Publ. Co. Inc., 1983, pp. 251-263.
46. Fernbach DJ, Donaldson M, Lane D, Lonsdale D, Vietti TJ: The treatment of advanced acute leukemia in children with concomitant vincristine sulfate and cyclophosphamide. In: Proceedings of the Twelfth International Society of Hematology, Jaffe ER (ed), New York, 1968, p. 8.
47. Frei E III, Karon M, Levin RH et al: The effectiveness of combinations of antileukemia agents in inducing and maintaining remission in children with acute leukemia. Blood 26:642-656, 1965.
48. Skipper HE, Schabel FM Jr, Wilcox WS: Experimental evaluation of potential anticancer agents. XIII. On the criteria and kinetics associated with curability of experimental leukemia. Cancer Chemother. Rep. 35:1-111, 1964.
49. Selawry OS (for Acute Leukemia Cooperative Group B): New treatment schedule with improved survival in childhood leukemia: Intermittent parenteral vs. daily oral methotrexate for maintenance of induced remission. JAMA 194:75-81, 1965.
50. Nagao T, Lampkin BC, Mauer AM: Maintenance therapy in acute childhood leukemia. J. Pediatr. 76:134-137, 1970.
51. Holland JF, Glidewell O: Complementary chemotherapy in acute leukemia. In: Recent Results in Cancer Research: Advances in the Treatment of Acute (Blastic) Leukemias, Mathe G (ed), New York, Springer-Verlag New York, Inc., 1970.
52. Australian Cancer Society's Childhood Leukemia Study Group: Cyclic drug regimen for acute childhood leukemia. Lancet 1:313-318, 1968.
53. Goldin A, Venditti JM, Humphreys SR et al: Modification of treatment schedules in the management of advanced mouse leukemia with amethopterin. J. Nat. Cancer Inst. 17:203-212, 1956.
54. Lewis B: Somatic Cell Mutants in Gene Expression, 2nd Ed., Lewis B (ed), John Wiley and Sons, New York, pp. 142-188.
55. Mauer AM: Cell kinetics and practical consequences for therapy of acute leukemia. N. Eng. J. Med. 293:389-393, 1975.
56. Saunders EF, Lampkin BC, Mauer AM: Variation of proliferating activity in leukemia cell populations of patients with acute leukemia. J. Clin. Invest. 46:1356-1363, 1967.
57. Gavosto F, Pileri A, Gabutti V et al: Unusual blast proliferation and kinetics in acute lymphoblastic leukaemia. Europ. J. Cancer 5:343-348, 1969.
58. Gavosto F, Pileri A, Peforaso L: Proliferative kinetics of acute leukemia cells in relation to the chemotherapy. Acta. Genet. Med. Gemellol. 17:30, 1968.

59. Karle H, Ernst P, Killman S: Changing cytokinetic patterns of human leukaemic lymphoblasts during the course of the disease, studied in vivo. Br. J. Haemat. 24:231-244, 1973.
60. Steel GG: Cell population kinetics of human tumors. In: Growth Kinetics of Tumors, Steel GG (ed), Clarendon Press, 1977, pp. 185-216.
61. Wagner HP, Cottier H, Cronletie EP: Variability of proliferative patterns in acute lymphoid leukemia of children. Blood 39:176-186, 1972.
62. Edelstein M, Valeriote F, Vietti T: Influence of continuous infusion of cytosine arabinoside on sequencing with daunorubicin in L1210 leukemia. Cancer Treat. Rep. 62: 547-548, 1978.
63. Pinkel D: Treatment of acute leukemia. Pediatr. Clin. North Am. 23:117-130, 1976.
64. Schabel FM Jr: In vivo leukemic cell kill kinetics and "curability" in experimental systems. In: The Proliferation and Spread of Neoplastic Cells, Baltimore, The Williams & Wilkins Co., 1968, pp. 379-408.
65. Skipper HE: Cellular kinetics associated with curability of experimental leukemias. In: Perspectives of Experimental Leukemias, Dameshek W, Dutcher RM (eds), New York, Grave and Stratton, Inc., 1968, pp. 187-215.
66. Skipper HE, Schabel FM et al: Implications of biochemical, cytokinetic, pharmacologic and toxicologic relationships in the design of optimal therapeutic schedules. Cancer Chemother. Rep. 54:431-450, 1970.
67. Pinkel D: Patterns of failure in acute lymphocytic leukemia. Cancer Treat. Symp. 2:259-266, 1983.
68. Freireich EJ, Henderson ES, Karon MR, Frei E III: The treatment of acute leukemia considered with respect to cell population kinetics. In: Proliferation and Spread of Neoplastic Cells, Baltimore, The Williams & Wilkins Co., 1968, pp. 441-452.
69. Henderson ES: Combination chemotherapy of acute lymphocytic leukemia of childhood. Cancer Res. 27:2570-2572, 1967.
70. George SL, Fernbach DJ, Vietti TJ et al: Factors influencing survival in pediatric acute leukemia: The SWCCSG Experience, 1958-1970. Cancer 32:1542-1553, 1973.
71. Evans AE: Central nervous system involvement in children with acute leukemia. Cancer 17:256-258, 1963.
72. Kuo AH-M, Yatagonas X, Galicich JH, Fried J, Clarkson BD: Proliferative kinetics of central nervous system (CNS) leukemia. Cancer 36:232-239, 1975.
73. Tsuchiya J, Mofelel M, Shimano S et al: Proliferative kinetics of the leukemia cells in meningeal leukemia. Cancer 42:1255-1262, 1978.
74. Johnson R: An experimental therapeutic approach to L1210 leuekmia in mice: Combination chemotherapy and central nervous system irradiation. J. Natl. Cancer Inst. 32: 1333-1341, 1964.

75. Simone JV: Factors that influence haematological remission duration in acute lymphocytic leukemia. Br. J. Haem. 32: 461-468, 1976.
76. Simone JV, Aur RJA, Hustu HO et al: Combined modality therapy of acute lymphocytic leukemia. Cancer 35:25-35, 1975.
77. Simone JV, Aur RJA, Hustu HO et al: Three to ten years after cessation of therapy in children with leukemia. Cancer 42:839-844, 1978.
78. Simone JV: Acute lymphocytic leukemia in childhood. Seminars in Hematology 11:25-39, 1974.
79. Haghbin M, Murphy ML, Tan CC et al: A long term clinical followup of children with acute lymphoblastic leukemia treated with intensive chemotherapy regimens. Cancer 46: 241-252, 1980.
80. Haghbin M: Chemotherapy of acute lymphoblastic leukemia in children. Am. J. Hematol. 1:201-209, 1976.
81. Haghbin M, Tan CC, Clarkson BD, Mike V, Burchenal JH, Murphy ML: Intensive chemotherapy in children with acute lymphoblastic leukemia (L-2 protocol). Cancer 33:1491-1498, 1974.
82. Haghbin M, Tan CTC, Clarkson BD, Mike V et al: Treatment of acute lymphoblastic leukemia in children with "prophylactic" intrathecal methotrexate and intensive systemic chemotherapy. Cancer Res. 35:807-811, 1975.
83. Sullivan MP, Chen T, Dyment PG et al: Equivalence of intrathecal chemotherapy and radiotherapy as central nervous system prophylaxis in children with acute lymphatic leukemia: A Pediatric Oncology Group Study. Blood 60:948-958, 1982.
84. Freeman AI, Brecher ML, Wang JJ et al: Intermediate dose methotrexate (IDM) in childhood acute lymphocytic leukemia (ALL). In: Modern Trends in Human Leukemia III, Neth R, Gallo RC, Hofschneider P-H et al (eds), Berlin, Springer-Verlag, 1979, p. 115.
85. Freeman AI, Weinberg V, Brecher ML et al: Comparison of intermediate-dose methotrexate with cranial irradiation for the post-induction treatment of acute lymphocytic leukemia in children. NEJM 308:477-484, 1983.
86. Green DM, Brecher ML, Blumenson LE et al: The use of intermediate dose methotrexate in increased risk childhood acute lymphoblastic leukemia: A comparison of three versus six courses. Cancer 50:2722-2727, 1982.
87. Nesbit ME, Sather H, Robison LL et al: Sanctuary therapy: A randomized trial of 724 children with previously untreated acute lymphoblastic leukemia: A report from the Children's Cancer Study Group. Cancer Res. 42:674-680, 1982.
88. Nesbit ME, Sather HN et al: Presymptomatic central nervous system therapy in previously untreated childhood acute lymphoblastic leukemias: Comparison of 1800 rad and 2400 rad. A report from the Children's Cancer Study Group. Lancet 1:461-465, 1981.

89. Sallan SE, Hitchcock S et al: Influence of intensive asparaginase in the treatment of childhood non T-cell acute lymphoblastic leukemia. Cancer Res. 43:5601-5607, 1983.
90. Capizzi RL: Schedule dependent synergism and antagonism between methotrexate and L-asparaginase. Biochem. Pharmacol. 23:151-162, 1974.
91. Krance R, Newman D et al: Intermediate dose methotrexate and arabinosyl cytosine in combination therapy of childhood acute lymphocytic leukemia. Proc. Amer. Assoc. Clin. Oncol. 20:201, 1984.
92. Amadori S, Papa G, Avvisati G et al: Sequential combination of systemic high-dose Ara-C and asparaginase for the treatment of central nervous system leukemia and lymphoma. J. Clin. Oncol. 2:98-101, 1984.
93. Zim S, Johnson CE, Chabner BA, Poplack DG: Cellular pharmacokinetics of 6-mercaptopurine in human leukemia and lymphoma cells. Proc. of Amer. Assoc. Cancer Res. 25:349, 1984.
94. Willoughby MLN: Treatment of overt meningeal leukemia in children: Results of second MRC meningeal leukemia trial. Br. Med. J. 1:864-867, 1976.

10

PROGNOSTIC FACTORS IN CHILDHOOD ACUTE LYMPHOBLASTIC LEUKEMIA: CORRELATION WITH TREATMENT RESPONSE

Y. Ravindranath, M.B., B.S.

In 1949 Dr. Zuelzer, in his note on progress in pediatric hematology, made a then passing observation that in childhood ALL, the level of WBC at diagnosis has a bearing on survival (1). He noted, in a group of children with leukemia treated before the days of chemotherapy, that those presenting with WBC 10,000 at diagnosis, survived longer than those presenting with higher WBC counts. Some nineteen years later in 1968, Hardisty and Till (2) observed that children with ALL presenting with mediastinal mass (ALL + MM) have a poor outcome and show distinctly different clinical characteristics and thus, may have a biologically different form of ALL compared to others. In a later study (3) we confirmed this and showed that children with ALL + MM tend to have higher WBC, higher hemoglobin and platelet counts at presentation; that this presentation is seen more often in boys of older age and that they relapse early and their survival is shorter. From these modest beginnings we have come a long way in recognizing that childhood ALL is a heterogeneous disease both in terms of clinical presentation and biologic characteristics. It is now well accepted that treatment has to be "tailored", keeping in mind the clinical prognostic factors and immunologic subtypes of ALL.

It is interesting to note that the early observations of Zuelzer, Hardisty and Till, and others, were not fully appreciated until survival was significantly improved by more effective methods of therapy. Two major advances account for most of the success achieved in the treatment of childhood ALL - the use of Vincristine (VCR) and Prednisone (Pred) as standard drugs during induction and the routine inclusion of Central Nervous System (CNS) prophylaxis in the management of childhood ALL.

1. IMMUNOLOGIC PHENOTYPES IN CHILDHOOD ALL, CORRELATION WITH HEMATOLOGIC FINDINGS AND OUTCOME.

In the past decade, numerous investigations have contributed to the immunologic characterization of childhood ALL and this has been discussed in earlier chapters. The first of these observations consist in the demonstration that lymphoblasts from patients with ALL with a mediastinal mass possess receptors for sheep erythrocytes - T-lymphocyte marker. Subsequently the use of hetero and monoclonal antisera have lead to the recognition of several distinct immunologic subtypes of childhood ALL. One such classification is presented in Table 1. It is now possible to correlate the immunophenotypes, clinical characteristics, and outcome. The most comprehensive of such correlative studies have come from the Pediatric Oncology Group (POG) (4).

TABLE 1

CLASSIFICATION OF A.L.L. BY IMMUNOLOGIC SURFACE MARKERS

T-Cell
E-rosette postive or anti-T positive

B-Cell
Surface immunoglobulin (sIg) positive

Pre B-Cell
sIg negative
Cytoplasmic immunoglobulin (cIg) positive

Common A.L.L.
Anti-Common A.L.L. Antigen (CALLA) positive
Anti-B ("Ia, HBLA, etc.) positive
E-rosette negative or anti-T negative
sIg negative
cIg negative

Undifferentiated
CALLA positive
Anti-B positive only

The definition of immunologic subtypes in the POG studies are as follows. B-cell ALL was defined as those cases with >10% surface immunoglobulin (sIg) positive blasts; pre-B cell ALL >40% pan T (pT) antigen positive blasts, and the remainder were classified as null cell ALL. The results of immunophenotype studies (carried out at the two reference laboratories for POG) are shown in Table 2. As can be seen, B-cell leukemia is extremely rare. T-cell leukemias account for 14% of all the cases of ALL. The rest fall into the null (sIg^-, cIg^-, T^-) or pre-B category (sIg^-, cIg^+, T^-). The clinical prognostic grouping is based on age and WBC at diagnosis (Table 3).

All this classification, obviously, has meaning only if differences in treatment response can be shown. In the POG studies where treatment was evaluated, the patients with the null and pre-B variants were treated as per POG 7865 ALinC 12 regimens and the majority of children with T-cell leukemia were treated by a modified LSA_2-L_2 regimen. In the ALinC 12 regimen induction therapy consisted of VCR + Pred + L-Asparaginase (L-Asp) in regimens 1 and 2, and VCR + Pred in regimen 3. Regimen 3 patients received consolidation therapy with Cyclophosphamide (CTX), L-Asp, Methotrexate (MTX). CNS prophylaxis in regimen 1 was with cranial radiation + Intrathecal (IT) meds x 5, and IT meds only in regimen 3. T-cell ALL patients were treated by a modified LSA_2-L_2 regimen (5). Induction was with VCR + Pred + Daunorubicin; consolidation with Cytosine arabinoside (Ara-C), 6-Thioguamine (6-TG), L-Asp, BCNU, and maintenance was with alternating drug pairs. Even with the more intensive regimen for induction, fewer children with T-cell leukemia attained remission compared to either null or pre-B subtypes (Table 4).

The significance of immunophenotype on the duration of remission and the significance of clinical prognostic features within the immunophenotypic subgroups as shown in Figures 1-3. As can be seen in Figure 1, T-cell patients fared poorly compared to the null patients, despite a more intensive consolidation and maintenance regimen. The major unexpected finding

TABLE 2

PEDIATRIC ONCOLOGY GROUP

GROUPING OF 311 PEDIATRIC PATIENTS WITH A.L.L.
USING sIg, cIg, E-ROSETTE
AND MEMBRANE ANTIGEN TESTING

	# PATIENTS	PERCENTAGE
NULL (sIg^-, cIg^-, pT^-, Thy^-, E^-)	209	67.2%
PRE-B (sIg^-, cIg^+, pT^-, Thy^-, E^-)	56	18.0%
B-CELL (sIg^+, cIg^-, pT^-, Thy^-, E^-)	2	0.6%
T-CELL (sIg^-, clg^-, pT^+, Thy^+ or Thy^-, E^+ or E^-)	44	14.1%

(From Pullen J, et al: NY Acad Sci, 1984, with permission)

TABLE 3

PEDIATRIC ONCOLOGY GROUP

DEFINITION OF ALinC 12 RISK GROUPS*

	AGE (year)				
FEATURE	1	1-2	3-5	6-10	10
WBC (per ul)					
<10,000	B	A	A	A	B
10,000 - 99,999	B	B	A	B	B
$\geq$100,000	B	B	B	B	B
Liver or spleen below umbilicus; significant extra-medullary disease	B	B	B	B	B

*A = good prognosis, B = poor prognosis
(From: Pullen J, et al: NY Acad Sci, 1984, with permission)

in the POG studies was the emergence of pre-B phenotypes as a poor prognostic feature. Pre-B patients did as poorly as the T-cell type and the difference between pre-B and null patients was highly significant, p being <0.002. More details of pre-B leukemia will be presented later. As has been noted by everyone else, B-cell leukemia carried the worst prognosis. Analysis of data by the clinical prognostic grouping continued to show the difference between the null and T subgroups. T-cell patients relapse more frequently within each prognostic group (Figure 2A). The same is true when the data are analyzed by WBC at diagnosis, a finding which confirms our early observations (Figure 2B) (3). What is interesting in this data, however, is the fact that the difference in CCR rates was greater in the good prognosis patients than in the poor prognosis patients - a finding that differs from the Children Cancer Study Group (CCSG) observation that within clinical prognostic groups, T-cell markers have no independent significance (6).

TABLE 4

PEDIATRIC ONCOLOGY GROUP

RESPONSE TO REMISSION INDUCTION THERAPY
COMPARISON OF IMMUNOLOGIC SUBGROUPS

	#(%) FAILED INDUCTION	#(%) DEATHS DURING INDUCTION	#(%) ATTAINED CR
NULL	7 (3.3%)	2 (1.0%)	200 (95.7%)
PRE-B	1 (1.2%)	0	83 (98.8%)
T	6 (7.9%)	3 (3.9%)	67 (88.2%)

% ATTAINING CR:

NULL vs PRE-B: P = .3 (NS)
T vs (PRE-B + NULL): P = .01

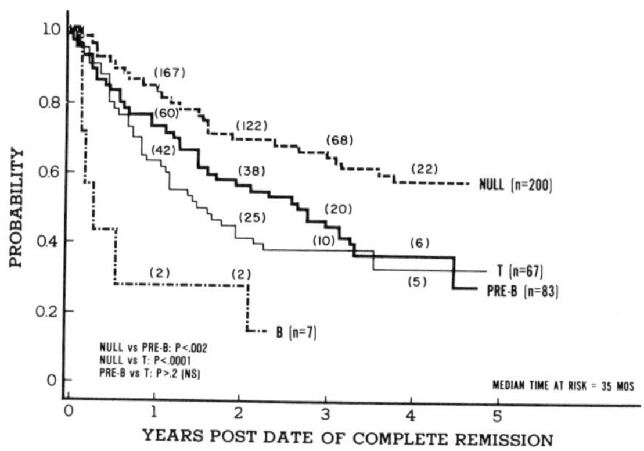

Figure 1. Duration of continuous complete remission (CCR) for the "null", pre-B, and T groups of patients with acute lymphocytic leukemia in the pilot ALinC 13 C study (POG 7865). Failure is defined as initial relapse at any site or death while in CCR. Patients who were lost to follow-up while still in CCR are considered censored observations. The number of patients who remain at various points in time are noted in parentheses. (From Pullen J, et al: NY Acad Sci 428:26, 1984, with permission).

Pre-B cell leukemia was first described by Vogler et al in 1978 (7) and is distinguished from B-cell leukemia by the presence of cytoplasmic Ig but no sIg. Pre-B leukemia was further characterized by the cooperative studies of POG and reported recently by Crist et al (8). Seventy-eight children with pre-B cell leukemia were analyzed (Table 5). There seems to be a slight excess of black children in the pre-B compared to the null group. In every other respect, pre-B cell leukemia is clinically and morphologically indistinguishable from null (non-T, non-B ALL) subgroup. Pre-B leukemia differs from T-cell ALL much the same way as the null subgroup except with regard to FAB morphology. As has been stated earlier, pre-B patients

(A)

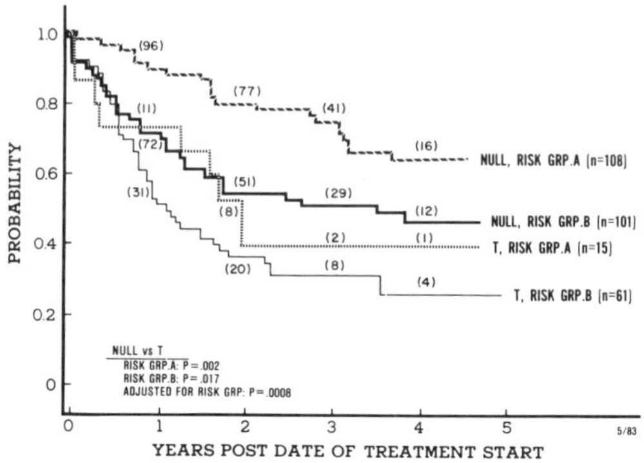

(B)

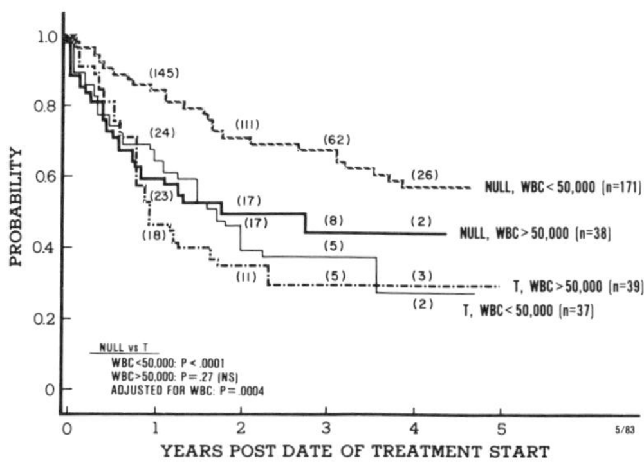

Figure 2. Time to initial treatment failure for the "null" and T groups of patients with acute lymphocytic leukemia in the pilot ALinC 13 C study by (A) distribution within risk groups A and B, (B) initial WBCs less than or greater than 50,000 ul. Failure is defined as induction failure, initial relapse at any site or death while in continuous complete remission (CCR). Patients who were lost to follow-up while still in CCR are considered censored observations. The median time at risk for patients continuing in CCR is 36 months. The number of patients who remain at risk at various points in time are noted in parentheses. (From: Pullen J, et al: NY Acad Sci 428:26, 1984, with permission).

relapsed more frequently compared to the null subgroup. This difference in the CCR rate was maintained even after adjustment for risk groups and WBC alone (Figures 3A, B).

(A)

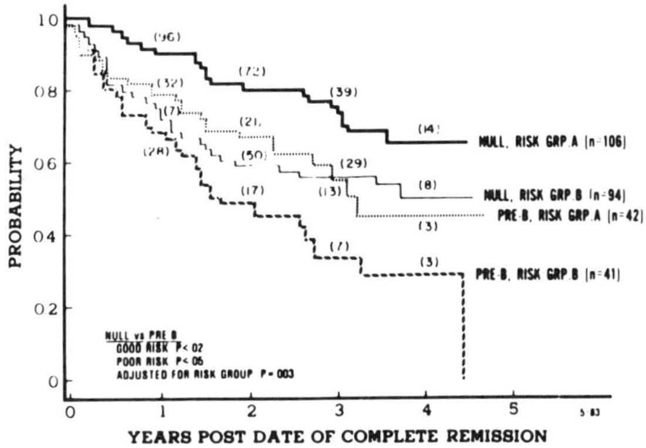

(B)

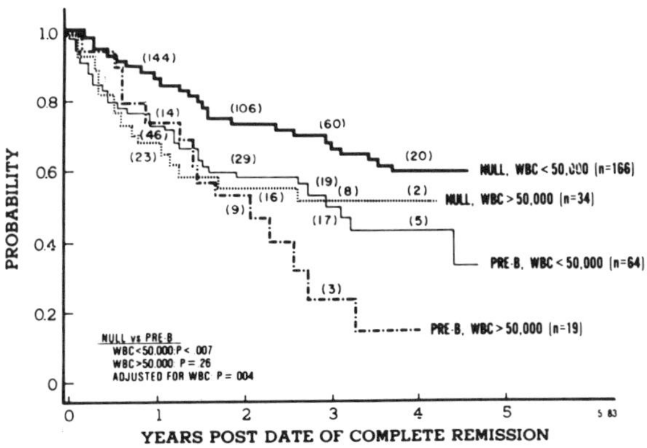

Figure 3. Duration of continuous complete remission (CCR) for the "null" and pre-B groups of patients with acute lymphocytic leukemia in the pilot ALinC 13 C study (POG 7865) by (A) distribution within risk groups A and B and (B) initial WBCs less than or greater than 50,000/ul. Failure is defined as initial relapse at any site or death while in CCR. Patients who were lost to follow-up while still in CCR are considered censored observations. The median time at risk for patients continuing in CCR is 35 months. The number of patients who remain at risk at various points in time are noted in parentheses. (From: Pullen J, et al: NY Acad Sci 428:26, 1984, with permission).

TABLE 5

PEDIATRIC ONCOLOGY GROUP

COMPARATIVE FEATURES OF A.L.L. SUBCLASSES

CHARACTERISTICS ANALYZED	PRE-B (n = 78)	"NULL" (n = 201)	T (n = 76)	p value PRE-B VERSUS "NULL"	p value T VERSUS "NULL" + PRE-B
Demographic					
Age (yr)[a]	4.3	4.4	7.4	NS[b]	<0.001
Sex (male:female)	1.1	1.3	2.0	NS	0.07
Race (white:black)	3.9	9.1	4.4	0.03	NS
Corporal					
Mediastinal mass (%)	1.3	0.5	38.2	NS	<0.001
White cells (10^9/liter)[a]	13.2	12.1	61.2	NS	<0.001
Platelets (10^9/liter)[a]	55.5	41.0	65.0	NS	<0.01
Cell phenotypic[c]					
FAB L 1 (%)	87.3	88.8	91.8	NS	NS
FAB L 2 (%)	11.3	9.4	4.9		
periodic acid-Schiff reactive (%)[d]	65.8	62.8	38.4	NS	<0.001
Acid phosphatase reactive (%)[d]	34.7	27.4	50.8	NS	<0.001
Ia (%)[d,e]	100.0	98.4	12.2	NS	<0.001
CALLA (%)[d,e]	94.0	89.0	15.3	NS	<0.001

[a] Expressed as median
[b] NS, no significant difference
[c] No L3 morphology was discovered (1.4% of slides were unsatisfactory for panel review and classification).
[d] Percent of patients who were positive
[e] Ia (and CALLA) testing was done on 50(50) per-B, 192(192) "null", and 74(72) T-cell leukemia patients.

(From: Crist W, et al: Blood 63:407, 1984, with permission)

Pullen et al analyzed the POG ALL data by both univariate and multivariate analysis. WBC, age and immunophenotype were the only other factors to be of prognostic significance independently. No other variables were of prognostic significance (Table 6). Within the null and pre-B subtypes, WBC and age were of significance (Table 7). Race was not a significant prognostic factor in the null, but was of significance in prognostication. Somewhat different conclusions were drawn by CCSG (6). Prominent lymphoadenopathy, hemoglobin level at diagnosis, sex and platelet count were also significant predictors of prognosis and interestingly thymic mass was not an independent prognostic variable.

TABLE 6

PEDIATRIC ONCOLOGY GROUP

RELATIONSHIP OF INITIAL CLINICAL OR LABORATORY FEATURES TO DURATION OF COMPLETE REMISSION. UNIVARIATE LIFE TABLE ANALYSIS OF THE COMBINED NULL + PRE-B GROUPS

CHARACTERISTIC	PROBABILITY	CHARACTERISTIC	PROBABILITY
WBC	<.0001	Platelet count	.15
Age	<.0001	Hepatomegaly	.65
Race	.03	Treatment	.59
Immunophenotype	.004	CNS Disease	.87
Hemoglobin	.09	Sex	.60
FAB	.15	Splenomegaly	.76

(From: Pullen J, et al: NY Acad Sci 428:26, 1984, with permission)

TABLE 7

PEDIATRIC ONCOLOGY GROUP

FACTORS PREDICTIVE OF DURATION OF CONTINUOUS COMPLETE REMISSION BY FORWARD STEP-WISE COX LIFE TABLE REGRESSION ANALYSIS. NULL GROUP ANALYZED SEPARATELY FROM PRE-B GROUP

VARIABLES OF INDEPENDENT SIGNIFICANCE*	DEGREES OF FREEDOM	CHI SQUARE	PROBABILITY
NULL			
WBC	1	14.1	<.001
Age	1	7.1	.008
PRE-B			
Sex	1	7.5	<.01
Age	1	5.6	.02
Race	1	4.6	.03

* Within each phenotype, variables are listed in order of entrance into model. No other variables tested were of independent significance.

(From: Pullen J, et al: NY Acad Sci 428:26, 1984, with permission)

2. SEX

In the past few years, much has been written about the prognostic implication of sex in childhood ALL (9,10). The poorer outcome in males noted in some studies was not due to the occurrence of testicular relapse as it has been previously shown by others that the difference between males and females persisted even after adjustment for testicular leukemia (9). As discussed earlier POG studies show that sex is a significant prognostic factor only within the pre-B subgroup, but not in the null or T-cell subtype (Table 7). In our studies at the Children's Hospital of Michigan, we did not see a significant difference in prognosis between sexes with regard to CCR (11). However, analysis of our data showed a higher incidence of CNS leukemia only among boys with high initial white counts (Table 8). In this particular study, interestingly, there were proportionately greater numbers of boys with high initial WBC compared to girls, even after the T-cell subgroup was excluded (11). An additional unique finding is that following cessation of therapy, sex is the only indicator of higher risk for relapse. Males relapse more frequently (12).

TABLE 8
CHILDREN'S HOSPITAL OF MICHIGAN
INCIDENCE OF CNS RELAPSE ON IMFRA CNS PROPHYLAXIS

	MALES	FEMALES	P VALUE	TOTAL
TOTAL	68	45		113
Number with CNS relapse	13	2	0.006	15 (13.3%)
WBC <20,000/ul	43	36		79
Number with relapse	4 (9.3%)	2 (5.6%)	0.23	6 (7.6%)
WBC >20,000/ul	25	9		34
Number with CNS relapse	9 (36%)	0	<0.001	9 (26.5%)

(Y. Ravindranath, et al.) (11)

3. COMMON ALL ANTIGEN (CALLA)

Several investigators have shown that CALLA negativity is associated with a poorer outcome (13,14,15). POG data did not confirm this but the data showed that the majority of infants under one year of age (an age group known to have poorer outcome) had CALLA negative blast cells (4). This appears to be a possible explanation for the poorer outcome associated with CALLA negativity. Whether within various age groups CALLA positivity or negativity will be independently significant is yet to be determined.

4. OTHER PROGNOSTIC VARIABLES

The immunosuppressive effects of leukemia itself have been shown to be predictive of prognosis. Low levels of IgG, IgA, IgM at diagnosis were found to be associated with poorer outcome (6). Finally, karyotype is emerging as an important predictor of outcome (16). Preponderance of hyperdiploid cells was associated with longer remission while pseudodiploidy with the poorest outcome. Patients with predominantly normal or hypodiploid cell lines had intermediate outcomes.

5. NEWER THERAPEUTIC APPROACHES

Based on these observations, several studies have been initiated in which therapy has been intensified for those presenting with high risk features such as high WBC count:T-cell ALL; age <2; >10; massive organomegaly and those with CNS disease at diagnosis (17,18,19). Complicated formulae have been developed by some investigators to distinguish low and high risk groups (20). Exact comparison of various studies is not possible because of differences in definitions of high risk features. Nonetheless, initial results of these studies suggest that intensification of therapy, particularily in the first 6 months of therapy, improves the results for children with "high risk" ALL. The studies that have attracted most attention are those of the BFM (Berlin-Frankfort-Munich) group in West Germany (17,18).

In the BFM 76/69 study, children presenting with high risk features were given intensive consolidation in the first six months following induction with dexamethasone, VCR, Adriamycin (Adr), L-Asp (for 4 weeks) followed by CTX, Ara-C, and 6-TG (for 2 weeks). CNS prophylaxis was with cranial irradiation. Current results show that the five year disease-free survival rate for all patients in the study was 69%. There was no difference in the CCR rate between low and high risk groups. The previously noted poorer outcome for those presenting with WBC >25,000; age <2; >10; and T-cell ALL were no longer evident. Thus, with a more aggressive treatment, the outcome in high risk category has been improved significantly.

Based on the premise that T-cell leukemia is biologically different from non-T, non-B ALL, we at the Children's Hospital of Michigan have initiated a new treatment program for T-cell ALL and limited entry into the study to those presenting with mediastinal mass (21). Remission induction was with VCR weekly times for 4 weeks, Adriamycin at day 1 and 21 and Pred daily x 3 weeks. This was followed by a 10 day course of L-Asp I.M. daily. Maintenance was with alternating cycles of VCR + Adr (week 1 only) + Pred for 3 weeks and IV MTX (30 mg/kg) at 3-4 week intervals x 4. CNS prophylaxis was with IT MTX x 4 during induction and with first and fourth IV MTX of the 4 dose IV MTX cycle. Total duration of therapy is 3 years. So far all patients have been entered on study, 9 achieved remission and 2 patients relapsed. Eight continue in remission from 6 months to 5 years with a median of 2 years. Three patients are off all therapy and doing well. These preliminary results are encouraging and suggest that prognosis will be improved in T-cell ALL patients with more intensive therapy.

At the same time as the treatment has been intensified for those with high risk features, studies have been designed to reduce therapy for those with low risk features. Following the initial reports from St. Jude Hosptial (22), with CNS prophylaxis with cranial radiation with +IT MTX x 5 has been widely adopted. At the same time, several different approaches to CNS prophylaxis have been developed by other investigators - intermittent IT MTX and fractional irradiation (IMFRA) (23); intermittent IT MTX alone (24); triple IT therapy (IT MTX-Ara-C, hydrocortisone) during induction and remission maintenance (25); and intermediate dose MTX (IDM) (26,27). In brief, these studies showed that several effective methods of CNS prophylaxis are available and the eventual superiority of one or the other regimen depends on the CNS toxicity associated with these regimens. Because of the toxicity associated with the so-called "standard" 2400 rad cranial radiation regimen, the Children's Cancer Study Group initiated a randomized trial comparing 1800 rad vs. 2400 rad cranial irradiation for CNS prophylaxis (28). The lower dose of cranial radiation was found to be equally effective. Subsequently, the same group compared IT MTX alone vs. 1800 rad cranial irradiation + IT MTX in low risk patients and found that IT MTX alone was effective in preventing CNS leukemia in low risk patients (29), thereby confirming the earlier observation of other investigators.

Thus therapy of childhood ALL has entered a new era, namely specific therapy for patients with differing risks for relapse. It is to be hoped that these efforts will lead to successful therapy for all children with leukemia.

ACKNOWLEDGEMENTS

The author thanks Dr. Jeannette Pullen, Dr. William Crist and Dr. Teresa Vietti for their help and advise in preparing this manuscript and for making available the data from Pediatric Oncology Group studies for presentation and publication. The author thanks Mrs. Julie Nucci for typing this manuscript.

REFERENCES

1. Zuelzer WW: Current trends in hematology. Pediatrics 4: 269, 1949.
2. Hardisty RM, Till MW: Acute leukemia 1959-1964: Factors affecting prognosis. Arch. Dis. Child. 43:107-115, 1969.
3. Ravindranath Y, Kaplan J, Zuelzer WW: Significance of mediastinal mass in acute lymphoblastic leukemia. Pediatrics 55:889-893, 1975.
4. Pullen DJ, Boyett JM, Crist W et al: Pediatric oncology group utilization of immunologic markers in the designation of acute lymphoblastic leukemia (ALL) subgroups. Influence on treatment response. NY Acad. Sci. 428:26-48, 1984.
5. Pullen DJ, Sullivan MP, Falletta JM et al: Modified LSA_2-L_2 treatment in 53 children with E-rosette-positive T-cell leukemia: Results and prognostic factors. Blood 60:1159-1168, 1982.
6. Miller DR, Leikin S, Albo V et al: Use of prognostic factors in improving the design and efficiency of clinical trials in childhood leukemia: Children's cancer group report. Cancer Treat. Rep. 64:381-392, 1980.
7. Vogler LB, Crist WM, Bockman DE et al: Pre B-cell leukemia. A new type of childhood lymphoblastic leukemia. N. Eng. J. Med. 298:872, 1978.
8. Crist W, Boyett J, Roper M et al: Pre B-cell leukemia responds poorly to treatment: A pediatric oncology group study. Blood 63:407-414, 1984.
9. Baumer J, Mott M: Sex and prognosis in childhood acute lymphoblastic leukemia. Lancet II:128-129, 1978.
10. Sather H, Miller DR, Nesbit M et al for the children's cancer study group: Differences in prognosis for boys and girls with acute lymphoblastic leukemia. Lancet I:739-743, 1981.
11. Ravindranath Y, Bhambhani K, Kelly JO et al: Central nervous system prophylaxis with intermittent intrathecal methotrexate and fractional radiation in childhood acute lymphoblastic leukemia. In: Central Nervous System Leukemia - Prevention and Treatment, Mastrangelo R, Poplack DG, Riccardi R (eds), Martinus Nijhoff, 1983.
12. George S, Aur RJA, Mauer A, Simone J: A reappraisal of the results of stopping therapy in childhood leukemia. N. Eng. J. Med. 300:269-273, 1979.
13. Greaves M, Janossy G, Peto J, Kay H: Immunologically defined subclasses of acute lymphoblastic leukemia in children: Their relationship to presentation features and prognosis. Brit. J. Haemat. 48:179-197, 1981.
14. Sallan SE, Ritz J, Pesando J et al: Cell surface antigens: Prognostic implications in childhood acute lymphoblastic leukemia. Blood 55:395-402, 1980.
15. Chessells JM, Hardisty RM, Rapson NT et al: Acute lymphoblastic leukemia in children: Classification and prognosis. Lancet II:1307-1309, 1977.

16. Secker-Walker LM, Lawler SD, Hardisty RM: Prognostic implications of chromosome findings in acute lymphoblastic leukemia at diagnosis. Br. Med. J. 2:1529-1530, 1978.
17. Henze G, Langermann HJ, Ritter J et al: Treatment strategy for different risk groups in childhood acute lymphoblastic leukemia: A report from the BFM study group. In: Haematology and Blood Transfusion: Modern Trends in Human Leukemia IV, Vol 26, Neth R, Gallo RC, Graf H (eds), Berlin, Springer-Verlag, 1981, p. 87.
18. Henze G, Lampert F, Langermann HJ et al: Prognosis of acute lymphoblastic leukemia related to initial findings and treatment. In: 13th International Cancer Congress, Part D, Research and Treatment, Alan R. Liss, New York, 1983, pp. 445-449.
19. Sallan SE, Hitchcock-Bryan S, Gelber R et al: Influences of intensive asparaginase in the treatment of childhood non-T acute lymphoblastic leukemia. Cancer Res. 43:5601-5607, 1983.
20. Palmer MK, Hann IM, Jones PM, Evans DI: A score at diagnosis for predicting length of remission in childhood acute lymphoblastic leukemia. Brit. J. Cancer 42:841-849, 1980.
21. Ravindranath Y. Unpublished observations.
22. Aur RJA, Simone JV, Hustu HO et al: Central nervous system therapy and combination chemotherapy lymphocytic leukemia. Blood 37:272-281, 1971.
23. Zuelzer WW, Ravindranath Y, Lusher JM et al: IMFRA (intermittent intrathecal methotrexate and fractional radiation) plus chemotherapy in childhood leukemia. Am. J. Hematol. 1:191-199, 1976.
24. Haghbin M, Murphy ML, Tan C et al: A long term clinical follow up of children with intensive chemotherapy regimens. Cancer (Phila)46:241-252, 1980.
25. Sullivan MP, Chen T, Dyment PG et al: Equilivalence of intrathecal chemotherapy and radiotherapy as central nervous system prophylaxis in children with acute lymphatic leukemia: A pediatric oncology group study. Blood 60: 948-958, 1982.
26. Freeman AI, Weinberg V, Brecher ML et al: Comparison of intermediate-dose methotrexate with cranial irradiation for the post induction treatment of acute lymphocytic leukemia in children. N. Eng. J. Med. 308:477-484, 1983.
27. Moe PJ, Seip M: High dose methotrexate in acute lymphocytic leukemia in childhood. Acta. Paediatr. Scand. 67: 265-268, 1978.
28. Nesbit ME Jr, Sather HN, Robison LL et al: Presymptomatic central nervous system therapy in previously untreated childhood acute lymphoblastic leukemia: Comparison of 1800 rad and 2400 rad. A report for children's cancer study group. Lancet I:461-466, 1981.
29. Coccia PF, Bleyer WA, Siegel SE et al for the Children's Cancer Study Group: Reduced therapy for children with good prognosis acute lymphoblastic leukemia. Blood 58:1372, 1981.

11

CLINICAL TRIALS IN ADULT ANLL: AN OVERVIEW

Michael Rooney, M.D.

Tremendous advances have been made over the past 20 years in the treatment of acute non lymphocytic leukemia (ANLL) in adults. This chapter will provide a historical perspective on the emergence of modern chemotherapy against ANLL. By reviewing past and current clinical trials, an appreciation of the stepwise progress which has been made in the understanding and management of this disease may be gained.

The recognition that long term survival for patients with ANLL was possible only if complete clinical and bone marrow remission were achieved, prompted the search for the most effective remission induction chemotherapy regimen. In the 1960's and early 1970's reports describing series of patients who received single agent chemotherapy, usually 6-mercaptopurine (6-MP), cytarabine (Ara-C), or daunorubicin (DNR) were published. These trials (Table 1) reported complete response rates between 12%-50% and identified Ara-C and the anthracycline antibiotic DNR as the most active single agents in adult ANLL. It was also during these trials that the dose response and scheduling characteristics of Ara-C were established in human subjects. In a Southwest Oncology Group study reported in 1974 (1), a 120 hour infusion of Ara-C at 1000 mg/m^2 resulted in a 38% complete response (CR) rate while a 48 hour infusion of 800 mg/m^2 resulted in 20% CR. The longer infusion time was chosen to expose leukemic blast cells to the drug for more than two generation times, a decision based on the S phase specificity of this chemotherapeutic agent. After dose adjustments in the second and subsequent courses, each treatment group was receiving essentially identical doses of Ara-C, establishing that schedule of administration and not dose was responsible for the differing response rates.

TABLE 1

SINGLE AGENT TRIALS IN ANLL

Published	Induction regimen	%CR	Ref
1960	6-MP	12	5
1968	6-MP	22	5
1974	Ara-C (800mg/m^2/dx2)	23	1
1974	Ara-C (1000mg/m^2/dx5)	40	1
1973	DNR (60mg/m^2/dx5)	43	3
1968	Ara-C (Various)	16	2
1972	DNR (60mg/m^2/dx3)	50	4
1975	Ara-C (100mg/m^2/d til hypoplasia)	14	6
1979	DNR (60mg/m^2/dx3)	48	7

The Acute Leukemia Group B (ALGB) studied the effectiveness of DNR given in a variety of schedules. In two trials involving untreated and previously treated patients published in 1973 (3), they showed that DNR given for 3 consecutive days at a dose of 60mg/m^2 was more effective (29% CR) than a 5 day (16% CR) or a 7 day (22% CR) regimen. The hematologic toxicity data from this study showed that the 7 day course of DNR was too toxic for most patients, and that only 50% of patients were able to tolerate 5 consecutive doses of DNR. A second ALGB study compared the same dose of DNR (60mg/m^2) given daily for 5 days versus twice weekly versus once weekly. In previously untreated adult patients, the 5 consecutive day treatment produced 43% CR, compared with 17% CR in each of the intermittent treatment arms. These scheduling trials were to lay important groundwork for subsequent combination chemotherapy regimens in ANLL.

The question of whether combination chemotherapy could offer improved complete response rates was addressed by several randomized trials in the 1970's which are summarized in Table 2. ALGB compared 4 treatment arms: Ara-C alone vs. Ara-C + 6-MP vs. Ara-C + 6 thioguanine (6-TG) vs. Ara-C + DNR. In this study, each of the 3 combination regimens was more effective at inducing complete remission than Ara-C alone (6). The Southwest Oncology Group (SWOG) conducted a randomized trial (12) comparing Ara-C vs. COAP in patients with acute leukemia and found that among adult patients with ANLL, 31% achieved CR status with Ara-C alone, vs. 45% of patients receiving COAP. The NCI conducted a randomized trial comparing DNR against a 4 drug regimen of DNR + Ara-C + 6-TG + pyrimethamine (8). The two regimens were equally effective with 49% and 46% CR rates respectively. Cancer and Leukemia Group B (CALGB) tested DNR alone against two combination regimens, Ara-C + 6-TG, and DAT (7) and found very similar CR rates with each induction program, 47%, 46%, and 50%, respectively. It is difficult to compare the results of these separate trials, but one may conclude from the above and from Table 2 that DNR given as a single agent is as effective as any combination chemotherapy induction program in these trials.

A large number of clinical trials have been conducted by single institutions and cooperative groups employing a wide variety of combination chemotherapy regimens in adult ANLL. Complete response rates after induction chemotherapy from a

Table 2

COMPARATIVE TRIALS; SINGLE AGENTS VS. COMBINATION CHEMOTHERAPY IN ANLL

Regimen	N	%CR	Ref
ALGB- 1974			
Ara-C 100mg/m^2 daily til hypoplasia	49	14	6
Ara-C as above + 6-MP 2.5mg/kg/d	56	27	
Ara-C as above + 6-TG 2.5mg/kg/d	66	36	
Ara-C as above + DNR 45mg/m^{2}x2	60	22	
SWOG- 1974			
Ara-C 200mg/m^2 day 1-5	51	31	12
CPM 100mg/m^2 day 1-5 VCR 2mg day 1 Ara-C 100mg/m^2 day 1-5 Prednisone 25mg qid day 1-5	57	45	
NCI- 1976			
DNR 60mg/m^2 day 1-3	33	49	8
DNR 75mg/m^2 day 1 Ara-C 75mg/m^2 q12hr day 1-5 6-TG 75mg/m^2 po q12hr day 1-5 Pyrimethamine 1mg/kg day 1-5	33	46	
CALGB-1979			
DNR 60mg/m^2 day 1-3	122	47	
Ara-C 100mg/m^2 q12hr til aplasia 6-TG 100mg/m^2 q12hr til aplasia	138	46	7
DNR 100mg/m^2 day 1 Ara-C 100mg/m^2 q12hr day 1-5 6-TG 100mg/m^2 q12hr day 1-5	129	50	

number of these trials are shown in Table 3. It becomes apparent that the most effective induction regimens contain some combination of DNR and Ara-C. The original "7+3" regimen reported by Holland and Yates (10) has been tested by others including CALGB and the Baltimore Cancer Research Center (BCRC) with similar high CR rates (Table 4). A study conducted at Roswell Park

Table 3

COMBINATION CHEMOTHERAPY INDUCTION PROGRAMS

	N	%CR	Ref.
1972- "L6"	43	65	9
Ara-C 3mg/kg q12hr til aplasia			
6-TG 2.5mg/kg q12hr			
1973- 7+3 (Holland & Yates)	16	63	10
Ara-C 100mg/m^2/dx7 by constant infusion			
DNR 45mg/m^2/d day 1-3			
1973- POMP	51	25	11
6-MP 500mg/m^2/dx5			
VCR 2mg day 1			
Methotrexate 7.5mg/m^2/dx5			
Prednisone 200mg/dx5			
1976- COAP	39	43	12
CPM 100mg/m^2/dx5			
VCR 2mg day 1			
Ara-C 100mg/m^2/dx5			
Prednisone 200mg/m^2/dx5			
1977- AcDAc (Hopkins)	25	56	13
Ara-C 45mg/m^2 day 1-2-3, 8-9-10			
DNR 1mg/kg/dx3			
1977- WCSG	55	28	14
Ara-C 100mg/m^2 q12hr til hypoplasia			
6-TG 80mg/m^2 q12hr			
1979- Roswell Park	36	66	15
7+3 ADR 30	46	71	15
10+3 ADR 30			
1979- VAPA	83	70	16
VCR 1.5mg day 1+5			
ADR 30mg/m^2 day 1-3			
Prednisone 40mg/m^2 q12hr day 1-5			
Ara-C 100mg/m^2/d by infusion x7			
1981- ROAP/AD-OAP	272	59	16a
ADR 40mg/m^2 or Rubidazone 200mg/m^2 day 1			
VCR 2mg day 1			
Prednisone 100mg/day day 1-5			
Ara-C 70-100mg/m^2/d x5-7			

Memorial Institute (15) attempted to improve on the results of 7+3 by extending the duration of the Ara-C infusion to 10 days, while employing a lower dose of anthracycline - in this case Doxorubicin (ADR) at 30mg/m^2 for 3 days. Although the 10+3 regimen resulted in a 71% CR rate compared with 66% CR for 7+3 (ADR 30mg/m^2/dx3), these differences were not statistically significant. More recently, the CALGB has attempted to define the optimal dose of anthracycline in the 7+3 style induction program. In a randomized trial comparing a 7 day infusion of Ara-C at 100mg/m^2/d combined with 3 different anthracycline components, DNR 30mg/m^2/dx3, DNR 45mg/m^2/dx3, and ADR 30mg/m^2/dx3, CR rates of 55%, 58%, and 50% were obtained, respectively. These differences were not statistically significant. Because a much higher incidence of gastrointestinal toxicity was noted in the group of patients randomized to the ADR arm, the authors reporting this study felt that DNR was the preferable anthracycline to use in combination with Ara-C. Frequency of response in patients over age 60 was greatest and treatment related morbidity and mortality lowest among the group receiving the lower dose of DNR, suggesting that less intensive therapy may be appropriate in this usually poor prognostic patient population.

Table 4

RESULTS IN ANLL WITH 7+3 INDUCTION CHEMOTHERAPY

Investigator	N	%CR	Ref.
Yates and Holland, 1973	16	65	10
CALGB, 1975	43	66	20
BCRC, 1979	60	60	21
CALGB, 1982			
7+3 DNR-45	226	58	22
7+3 DNR-30	213	55	
7+3 ADR-30	214	50	

Another induction regimen which has been widely tested is the 3 drug combination of DNR + Ara-C + 6-TG (Table 5). Very high complete remission rates have been attributed to this drug combination in single institution trials, suggesting that the addition of the third drug, 6-TG, is of benefit. In a randomized trial by the CALGB (28) which compared 3 induction regimens; 7+3, 10+3, and DAT, CR rates of 55%, 56%, and 57%, respectively were noted. The value of adding 6-TG to combinations of Ara-C and DNR has not been proven.

The next aspect of ANLL management to be addressed is that of post induction therapy. It is estimated that 10^8-10^9 viable leukemic cells exist in patients who have achieved CR; that is, patients with normocellular bone marrow containing fewer than 5% blasts who have normal peripheral WBC and platelet counts, and normal hemoglobin. By reducing this persistent population of leukemic cells further, duration of CR should be extended. This, of course, is the strategy behind consolidation, maintenance and late intensification chemotherapy in ANLL.

Table 5

RESULTS IN ANLL WITH DAUNORUBICIN, CYTARABINE AND THIOGUANINE.

	N	%CR	Ref
Lewis, 1983			
DNR 135mg/m^2 by 72hr infusion	19	60	17
Ara-C 100mg/m^2/dx10			
6-TG 100mg/m^2 q12hr day 3-10			
CALGB, 1979			
DNR 100mg/m^2 day 1	154	50	7
Ara-C 100mg/m^2 q12hr day 1-5			
6-TG 100mg/m^2 q12hr day 1-5			
Gale, 1977			
DNR 60mg/m^2/d days 5-7	28	79	18
Ara-C 100mg/m^2 q12hr day 1-7			
6-TG 100mg/m^2 q12hr day 1-7			
Rees, 1977			
DNR 50mg/m^2 day 1	20	85	19
Ara-C 100mg/m^2 q12hr day 1-5			
6-TG 100mg/m^2 q12hr day 1-5			

The results of numerous clinical trials employing a spectrum of maintenance therapy that ranges from no post induction treatment to extremely complex and intensive multi-drug regimens have been published. The controversy over the role of maintenance chemotherapy in ANLL can be illustrated by comparing the results of 5 trials for which long term follow-up data is available. Table 6 summarizes the treatment plans employed in these studies. At one extreme is the report from Champlin et al (23) describing 26% of complete responders in continuous CR at 5 years following induction and consolidation chemotherapy only, with no maintenance program at all. At the other extreme is the data from the VAPA protocol which describes 27% of patients who achieved CR remaining in continuous remission for 5 years after an 18 month course of intensive maintenance therapy consisting of 4 cycles of "induction strength" chemotherapy (26). It is interesting to note that this intensive maintenance regimen extends the median duration of remission to 27 months, yet fails to eliminate the risk of late relapse.

The maintenance therapy employed by CALGB study 7721, by Peterson and Bloomfield at the University of Minnesota, and by Gale, Foon, and associates at UCLA falls somewhere in between the two extremes mentioned above. The maintenance arms of these 3 trials vary in intensity, and are continued for 2-5 years after documentation of CR status. Median durations of remission are 12, 17, and 13 months with 20%-23% of complete responders enjoying long term continuous remission (22,24,25). From the results of these studies as well as others, it seems clear that only a minority of patients who achieve CR after induction therapy are potentially cured, and that the optimal post induction management of these patients has not yet been clearly defined.

The technique of allogeneic bone marrow transplantation for patients in remission represents in a sense the ultimate consolidation therapy, effectively eliminating, if successful, both malignant and normal stem cells. Approximately 80% of bone marrow transplant recipients remain in long term CR. Other

Table 6

RESULTS OF VARIOUS MAINTENANCE PROGRAMS IN ANLL

Induction	Consolidation	Maintenance	%CR	CR Med. Duration	Percent Relapse Free Remission	Ref.
DNR, Ara-C, 6-TG	AZA, ADRx1 DNR, Ara-C, 6-TGx1	None	62	14 mos	26(5yr)	1
DNR, Ara-C vs. ADR, Ara-C	None	2-3 yrs Ara-C + 1. 6-TG 2. Pred 3. DNR 4. Pred	55	12 mos	20(4yr)	2
Various	None	6-TG, Ara-C 5 years	58	17 mos	23(5yr)	3
DNR, Ara-C, 6-TG	DNR, Ara-C 6-TG	Ara-C, 6-TG, DNR $\pm$ IM for 2 years	82	13 mos	20(4yr)	4
VCR, ADR, Pred, Ara-C	See Below for maintenance schedule		70	27 mos	27(5yr)	5

AZA=5-azacytidine, ADR=Doxorubicin, Pred=Prednisone, Ara-C=Cytosine arabinoside, 6-TG=6-Thioguanine, DNR=Daunorubicin, VCR=Vincristine, IM=Immunotherapy

VAPA MAINTENANCE CHEMOTHERAPY

Sequence I	Sequence II	Sequence III	Sequence IV
ADR 45mg/m^2 day 1	ADR 30mg/m^2 day 1	VCR 1.5mg/m^2 day 1	Ara-C 200mg/m daily x 5 by infusion
Ara-C 200mg/m^2/d day 1-5 by infusion	AZA 150mg/m^2/d day 1-5 by infusion	Methylprednisolone 800mg/m^2/dx5 iv	
		6-MP 500mg/m^2/dx5	
		Mtx 7.5mg/m^2/dx5	
Given 4x at 3-4 wk intervals	Given 4x at 4 wk intervals	Given 4x at 3 wk intervals	Given 4x at 3-4 wk intervals

complications of bone marrow transplantation, most notably graft versus host disease and interstitial pneumonitis reduce the 5 year survivorship to approximately 60%, still comparatively better than conventional induction plus consolidation and/or maintenance chemotherapy programs in adult patients. If patients are stratified to age above and below 30, this survival advantage is found to apply only to patients less than age 30 (28). A prospective controlled single institution study at UCLA compared two groups of patients with newly diagnosed ANLL who received induction therapy composed of "TAD" for 1-3 courses (29). Patients who had HLA matched sibling donors went on to allogeneic bone marrow transplant. Forty-four patients with no available marrow donor received consolidation chemotherapy consisting of 1 course of AZA plus ADR followed by 1 course of TAD. Neither group received maintenance chemotherapy. Actuarial relapse and survival data are shown in Table 7. The similar 3 year survival statistics despite improved remission duration for the transplanted group illustrates the point that the role of bone marrow transplantation in adult patients with ANLL remains to be clearly defined. SWOG is currently conducting a prospective clinical trial of maintenance chemotherapy vs. bone marrow transplantation in adult ANLL similar to the UCLA study.

Allogeneic bone marrow transplantation is also being employed with some success in patients with relapsed or refractory ANLL. The Seattle transplant program has previously reported a 15% long term survivorship in such patients. In an attempt to improve the results of allogeneic bone marrow transplantation in this group of patients, the investigators at Wayne State University employed a sequential administration of high dose Ara-C for initial cytoreduction. After patients recovered from the acute toxicities of this treatment, cyclophosphamide and total bone marrow irradiation were then administered followed by allogeneic bone marrow transplantation. In a small pilot study of 6 patients with relapsed ANLL, 4 patients achieved a marrow remission after high dose Ara-C. All patients subsequently underwent allograft, and 4 remained in CR at 139, 80, 56, and 17 weeks post-transplant (30). These early results give rise to the hope that an improved cytoreductive regimen for refractory ANLL may be possible without prohibitive toxicity, resulting in improved long-term survival.

Table 7

BONE MARROW TRANSPLANT VS. CONSOLIDATION CHEMOTHERAPY IN ANLL

Regimen	N	Actuarial % Relapse free at 3 yr	Actuarial % Survival at 1 yr	Actuarial % Survival at 3 yr
Induction + BMT	33	22	59	43
		p=0.01		p=0.78
Induction + Consolidation	44	63	45	37

"TAD" Induction: Ara-C and 6-TG $100mg/m^2$ q12hr days 1-7
DNR $60mg/m^2$ days 5,6,7

Consolidation: 1. AZA $150mg/m^2/dx5$ by infusion
ADR $45mg/m^2/d$ day 4,5.

2. TAD as above for 1 course.

Attempts at prolonging duration of remission by employing various forms of immunotherapy have been included in many clinical trials in ANLL. Nonspecific immune stimulation has been attempted with agents such as Calmette-Guerin Bacillus, Corynebacterium Parvum and levamisole. Specific immunization with leukemia cells, cell free extracts and cultured cell lines has also been tried. The effect of immunotherapy on duration of remission has been inconsistent (Table 8) and there is little convincing data that immunotherapy is of benefit in the treatment of patients with ANLL.

Table 8

IMMUNOTHERAPY TRIALS IN ANLL

Center (Ref.)	N	Chemo- therapy	Immuno- therapy	Median Duration of CR (wks)	Remarks
Mt. Sinai Hosp.	70	+	-	24	
		+	+	88	Neuraminidase treated leuk. cells
		+	+	44	Neuraminidase treated leuk. cells + MER
Leukemia Group of Central Sweden	42	+	-	23	
		+	+	66	Calmette-Guerin bacillus + leuk. cells
Saint Bartholomews-Royal Marsden Hospital	5	+	-	28	
		+	+	44	Calmette-Guerin bacillus + leuk. cells
Medical Research Council	71	+	-	28	
		+	+	36	Calmette-Guerin bacillus + leuk. cells
M.D. Anderson	47	+	-	52	
		+	+	85	Calmette-Guerin bacillus
Hospital Edouard Herriot	63	+	-	52	
		+	+	65	Calmette-Drin bacillus
BCRC	60	+	-	25	
		+	+	23	Levamisole
Argentine Group for Treatment of AL	80	+	-	32	
		+	+	20	Corynebacterium p.
UCLA	47	+	-	77	
		+	+	56	Corynebacterium p. and leuk. cells
Albert Einstein University of Maryland (31)	50	+	-	104	
		+	+	96	Neuraminidase treated leuk. cells

Any review of clinical trials in ANLL must be undertaken with the understanding that varied and non-homogenous patient populations are being compared. In addition, the improvement in medical support capabilities for patients being treated for ANLL has resulted in improved remission and survival statistics for later trials irrespective of the chemotherapy program involved. Clear-cut prognostic indicators have been identified, including age >60 years at time of presentation, presence of cytogenetic abnormalities, pre-leukemic syndromes, and secondary leukemia, which greatly alter the likelihood of remission. These factors and their frequency in patient populations involved in clinical trials must be taken into account when comparing results from such trials.

Drs. E.J. Freireich and E.A. Gehan have employed the statistical technique of stepwise forward regression analysis to predict the likelihood of response in an individual patient based on pre-treatment clinical, cytogenetic, and biochemical parameters (32). This technique can be used to compare data from previous trials, as well as to design new chemotherapy trials more efficiently. The Intergroup Leukemia Study has been organized by Dr. Harvey Preisler at Roswell Park to concentrate efforts aimed at identifying factors which will predict for response in patients with ANLL.

Clinical trials of new chemotherapeutic agents in patients with relapsed ANLL have identified one promising agent with definite activity in this disease. Amsacrine (AMSA) used as a single agent at a variety of doses has produced CR in 17%-31% of patients with relapsed ANLL. Table 9 shows response data from trials in which AMSA is combined with other drugs. A recent ECOG pilot study of AMSA 100mg/m^2/dx3 and Ara-C 3gm/m^2 q12hr x 7 days resulted in a CR rate of 60% in previously untreated patients (33). The hepatotoxicity associated with this agent may limit its clinical usefullness, however its lack of cardiotoxicity makes it a promising replacement for anthracycline components in patients at risk for cardiac complications. As more trials including AMSA in first line therapy are completed, the role of this agent in the treatment of ANLL will be determined.

Table 9

AMSA COMBINATION CHEMOTHERAPY FOR ANLL

AMSA Dose mg/m^2/course	Other Agents mg/m^2	N	%CR	Ref.
600-740	Ara-C 200/dx5 6-TG 100 q12hr x10	25	32	34
210	Ara-C 70/d x7 VCR 2/d x1 Pred 100/d x5	56	46	35
750	AZA 150/d x5	14	50	36
675	VP16 200/d x3 Ara-C 200/d x3 6-TG 100-200/d x3	17	53	37
225-300	Ara-C 3000 q12hr x12	15	67	38
*300	Ara-C 3000 q12hr x14	30	60	33

* previously untreated patients

Ara-C, though not a new drug in the treatment of ANLL is receiving renewed attention in clinical trials at doses 30-fold higher than those used in conventional regimens. High dose Ara-C at $3gm/m^2$ q12hrx12 plus DNR $30mg/m^2$ on days 7-9 has been shown to overcome Ara-C resistance in 50% of patients with ANLL in relapse (39). Based on this experience, Wolf and associates at Vanderbilt have treated 27 adult patients with ANLL using standard induction regimens followed by 1-3 courses of high dose Ara-C ± DNR consolidation therapy. They report a median continuous CR duration of >31 months for this group of patients, with actuarial 4 year continuous remission projected at 56% (40). The CALGB is now conducting a cooperative study of high dose Ara-C intensification in ANLL.

Acute nonlymphocytic leukemia continues to foster active research at both basic science and clinical trial levels. As a result of the advances made over the past 20 years, a minority of patients can now hope to be cured of this once inevitably fatal illness. There is reason to be optimistic that further developments will convert this minority into a majority.

REFERENCES

1. Freireich EJ et al: Cytarabine for acute leukemia in adults. Arch. Inter. Med. 133:251-259, 1974.
2. Ellison RR et al: Arabinosyl cytosine: A useful agent in the treatment of acute leukemia in adults. Blood 32:507-523, 1968.
3. Weil M, Glidewell OJ, Jaquillat C: Daunorubicin in the therapy of acute granulocytic leukemia. Cancer Res. 33: 921-928, 1973.
4. Wiernik PH, Serpick AA: A randomized clinical trial of daunorubicin and a combination of prednisone, vincristine, 6-mercaptopurine and methotrexate in adult nonlymphocytic leukemia. Cancer Res. 32:2023-2026, 1972.
5. Boggs DR: The kinetics of neutrophilic leukocytes in health and disease. Semin. Hematol. 4:359-386, 1967.
6. Carey RW et al: Comparative study of cytosine arabinoside therapy alone and combined with thioguanine, mercaptopurine or daunorubicin in acute myelocytic leukemia. Cancer 36: 1560-1566, 1975.
7. Wiernik PH, Glidewell OJ et al: A comparative trial of daunorubicin, cytosine arabinoside, and thioguanine and a combination of the three agents for the treatment of acute myelocytic leukemia. Med. Ped. Onc. 6:261-277, 1979.
8. Weirnik PH, Schimpff SC et al: Randomized clinical comparison of daunorubicin alone with a combination of daunorubicin, cytosine arabinoside, 6-thioguanine and pyrimethamine for the treatment of acute nonlymphocytic leukemia. Cancer Treat. Rep. 60:41-53, 1976.
9. Clarkson BD: Acute myelocytic leukemia in adults. Cancer 30:1572-1582, 1972.

10. Yates JW, Holland JF et al: Cytosine arabinoside and daunorubicin therapy in acute nonlymphocytic leukemia. Cancer Chem. Rep. 57(4):485-488, 1973.
11. Rodriguez V, Hart JS, Freireich EJ et al: POMP combination chemotherapy of adult acute leukemia. Cancer 32:69-75, 1973.
12. Bodey GP, Coltman CA et al: Chemotherapy of acute leukemia. Arch. Intern. Med. 133:260-266, 1974.
13. Vaughan WP, Karp JE, Burke PJ: Long chemotherapy-free remissions after single cycle timed sequential chemotherapy for acute myelocytic leukemia. Cancer 45:859-865, 1980.
14. Lewis JP, Linman JW et al: Randomized clinical trial of cytosine arabinoside and 6-thioguanine in remission induction and consolidation of adult nonlymphocytic acute leukemia. Cancer 39:1387-1396, 1977.
15. Preisler H, Bjornsson S et al: Remission induction in acute nonlymphocytic leukemia: Comparison of a seven-day and ten-day infusion of cytosine arabinoside in combination with adriamycin. Med. Ped. Onc. 7:269-275, 1979.
16. Weinstein HJ, Mayer RJ et al: Treatment of acute myelogenous leukemia in children and adults. NEJM 303:473-478, 1980.
16a. Keating MJ, Smith TL et al: Four-year experience with anthracycline, cytosine arabinoside, vincristine and prednisone combination chemotherapy in 325 adults with acute leukemia. Cancer 47:2779-2788, 1981.
17. Lewis JP, Meyers F et al: Continuous infusion daunomycin in remission induction of acute nonlymphocytic leukemia. Blood 62:205a, 1983.
18. Gale RP, Cline MJ: High remission induction rate in acute myeloid leukemia. Lancet (1):497-499, 1977.
19. Rees JKH, Sandler RM et al: Treatment of acute myeloid leukemia with a triple cytotoxic regime: DAT. Br. J. Cancer 36:770-776, 1977.
20. Rai KR, Holland JF, Glidewell OJ: Improvement of remission induction of acute myelocytic leukemia. Proc. ASCO 16:265, 1975.
21. Chang P, Wiernik PH, Reich SD et al: Prediction of response to cytosine arabinoside and daunorubicin in acute nonlymphocytic leukemia. In: Therapy of Acute Leukemias, Mandelli (ed), Rome, Italy, Lombardo Editore, 1979, pp. 430-433.
22. Yates J, Glidewell OJ, Wiernik PH et al: Cytosine arabinoside with daunorubicin or adriamycin for therapy of acute myelocytic leukemia: A CALGB study. Blood 60:454-462, 1982.
23. Champlin R, Jacobs A, Gale RP et al: Prolonged survival in acute myelogenous leukemia without maintenance chemotherapy. Lancet (in press).
24. Peterson BA, Bloomfield CD: Long term disease free survival in acute nonlymphocytic leukemia. Blood 57:1144-1147, 1981.

25. Gale RP, Foon KA et al: Intensive chemotherapy for acute myelogenous leukemia. Annals Int. Med. 94:753-757, 1981.
26. Weinstein HJ, Mayer RJ et al: Chemotherapy for acute myelogenous leukemia in children and adults: VAPA update. Blood 62:315-319, 1983.
27. Preisler H, Kirshner J, Raza A, Davis R: Comparison of 3 remission induction regimens for the treatment of acute nonlymphocytic leukemia. Blood 62:206a, 1983.
28. Preisler H, Anderson K et al: Comparison of survival of patients with acute nonlymphocytic leukemia receiving maintenance chemotherapy or bone marrow transplantation in 1st remission. Proc. ASCO 2:177, 1983.
29. Champlin R, Zighelboim W et al: Treatment of acute myelogenous leukemia - bone marrow transplantation vs. consolidation chemotherapy. Proc. ASCO 2:180, 1983.
30. Foon KA, Gale RP: Controversies in the therapy of acute myelogenous leukemia. Amer. J. Med. 72:963-979, 1982.
31. Dutcher JP, Markus S, Wiernik PH et al: Intensive maintenance therapy in acute nonlymphocytic leukemia. Blood 62:201a, 1983.
32. Freireich EJ, Keating MJ, Gehan EA et al: Therapy of acute myelogenous leukemia. Cancer 42:874-882, 1978.
33. Hines JD, Oken MM, Mazza J et al: High dose cytosine arabinoside and M-AMSA induction and consolidation in acute nonlymphocytic leukemia. Blood 62:203a, 1983.
34. Arlin ZA, Flomenberg N et al: Treatment of acute leukemia in relapse with AMSA in combination with cytosine arabinoside and thioguanine. Cancer Clin. Trials 4:317-321, 1981.
35. McCredie KB, Keating MJ, Estey EH et al: Use of AMSA, cytosine arabinoside, vincristine, prednisone combination in poor risk patients in acute leukemia. Proc. AACR 22:479, 1981.
36. Kahn SB, Conroy JF, Bulova S et al: AMSA and 5-azacytidine therapy of acute leukemia. Blood 58:143a, 1981.
37. Hurd DD, Peterson BA, Bloomfield CD: AMSA, VP-16, cytosine arabinoside, and 6-thioguanine in the treatment of relapsed and refractory acute nonlymphocytic leukemia. Blood 58: 142a, 1981.
38. Hines JD, Oken MM, Mazza J et al: High dose cytosine arabinoside and AMSA in refractory acute nonlymphocytic leukemia. Blood 58:142a, 1981.
39. Herzig RH, Wolff SN, Karanes C et al: High dose cytosine arabinoside therapy for refractory leukemia. Blood 62: 361-369, 1983.
40. Wolff SN: High dose cytosine arabinoside and daunorubicin for acute nonlymphocytic leukemia in first remission. Proc. ASCO 25: 1984 (in press).

12

ALLOGENEIC MARROW TRANSPLANTATION FOR ACUTE NONLYMPHOBLASTIC LEUKEMIA IN ADULTS

Frederick R. Appelbaum, M.D. and E. Donnall Thomas, M.D.

1. INTRODUCTION

Over the past decade, marrow transplantation has progressed from a very experimental approach applied only to a handful of endstage leukemic patients to an important therapeutic option appropriate for many patients. In this paper we will describe the role marrow transplantation plays in the treatment of acute nonlymphoblastic leukemia (ANL) in adults. In order to define this role, the outcome of marrow transplantation obviously must be compared to that of more conventional chemotherapy for specific patient groups at given stages of their disease. Such comparisons are best made in prospective studies but only a few such studies have been performed and completed. For many patient groups only retrospective comparisons are possible. Retrospective analyses are inherently flawed and serve only as estimates. For some patient groups not even retrospective comparisons are possible because adequate data are not available.

The vast majority of clinical experience is derived from transplants using HLA-identical family members, and this review will consider only these patients. Our early experience with patients transplanted from donors mismatched at a single HLA locus (A, B, or D) suggests that they behave similarly to recipients of HLA-identical marrow (1). Experience with the use of family members mismatched for more than one antigen is very limited. Likewise, far too few patients have been transplanted using unrelated donors or autologous marrow to allow for any conclusions concerning these forms of transplantation.

Most of the transplant studies referred to in this review have used the "standard" Seattle preparative regimen which includes high-dose cyclophosphamide, 60 mg/kg on each of 2 days, followed by total body irradiation (TBI) delivered at 5-8 rad/min to a total dose of at least 1000 rad (2). A number of variations on the basic cyclophosphamide-TBI preparative regimen have been developed but there is as yet little evidence that these changes have had a major impact on the outcome of transplantation (3,4). Recently regimens that do not use TBI have been developed but, again, there is inadequate information to judge whether these regimens will change results (5).

Finally, patients included in the transplant studies have almost always been less than 50 years of age. This age limitation is arbitrary but is based on the general experience that the outcome of allogeneic marrow transplantation is less favorable in older individuals owing largely to an increased incidence and severity of graft-versus-host disease in older patients.

2. COMPARISON OF MARROW TRANSPLANTATION TO CHEMOTHERAPY

2.1 General considerations

If the goal of treatment of ANL is cure, then any comparison between marrow transplantation and chemotherapy must be based on results demonstrating long-term disease-free survival after therapy is stopped. For marrow transplantation there is excellent evidence that disease-free survival beyond 4 years from transplantation can be considered essentially equivalent to cure. Figure 1 is a Kaplan-Meier product limit estimates of the probability of being in remission for all 792 patients treated in Seattle with allogeneic marrow transplantation for acute leukemia (both ANL and acute lymphoblastic leukemia (ALL)) between December 1971 and January 1984. As shown, virtually all relapses had occurred by day 1500 after transplant. Thereafter only one relapse was seen among 53 patients alive and disease-free from 4 to 13 years after transplant. A second patient, not shown as relapsing in the curve, was transplanted for relapsed ALL and developed ANL in donor cells 6 years after transplantation. The fact that transplantation results in a virtual plateau in disease-free survival is an important point. Whether chemotherapy for ANL results in a similar plateau is less clear. Although several studies have documented that the relapse rate decreases significantly around 2 years after achieving complete remission (CR), relapses continue to be seen and there remains considerable debate about whether a true plateau in disease-free survival is ever achieved (6,7).

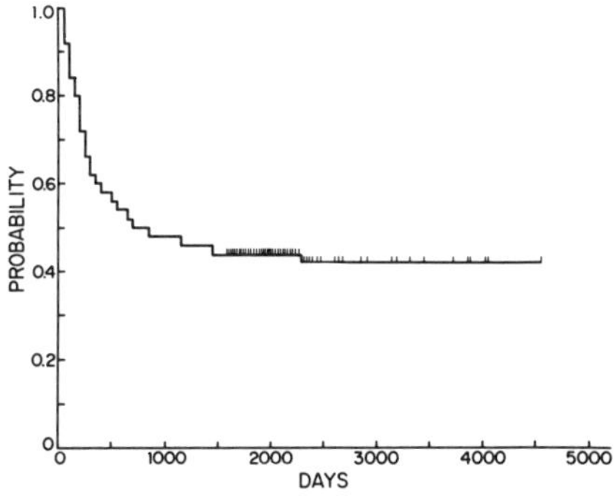

Figure 1. Kaplan-Meier product limit estimates of the probability of being in remission for all 792 patients treated in Seattle with allogeneic marrow transplantation for acute leukemia (both ANL and ALL) between December 1971 and January 1984. Ticks indicate patients alive and in remission beyond day 1550 from transplant.

Both transplantation and continued aggressive chemotherapy are associated with significant acute toxicities. Late life-threatening toxicities associated with chemotherapy are unusual but following transplantation there is the possibility that some patients will develop chronic graft-versus-host disease which can be disabling and life-threatening. Therefore, in comparing long-term results of chemotherapy and marrow transplantation, attention should be given not only to survival but to performance as well.

2.2 Refractory ANL

Patients who fail to achieve a first complete remission and those who relapse and fail to achieve a subsequent remission using standard chemotherapeutic regimens (such as anthracycline plus cytosine arabinoside) have an extremely poor prognosis with conventional or experimental chemotherapy. Although a small minority of such patients may respond completely to second or third line regimens or to experimental drugs, such responses are usually brief and virtually none of these patients can be cured with chemotherapy. Between 1970 and 1975, 54 patients with refractory ANL were transplanted from HLA-identical siblings and 6 are living and well 9-12 years after grafting with no further antileukemic therapy (8,9). Patients transplanted for refractory ANL are generally in poor physical condition at the time of transplantation and so have an increased chance of dying of nonleukemic causes during the transplant procedure. However, the major cause of treatment failure in this group is leukemic recurrence. Based on actuarial analyses, 65% of these patients either relapsed or would have relapsed had they not died of nonleukemic causes. Nonetheless, 10 to 15% of endstage patients can be cured with marrow transplantation. Since such patients have no other prospect for cure, marrow transplantation should be considered if facilities and an appropriately matched donor are available and if the patient is in reasonable clinical condition.

2.3 ANL in second remission or first relapse

Transplantation earlier, before patients have endstage refractory disease, allows for treatment while patients are in better clinical condition and, perhaps, before the leukemia has had a chance to acquire increased resistance to chemotherapy and radiotherapy. In Seattle, a group of 24 patients with ANL in second remission underwent allogeneic marrow transplantation (10). Kaplan-Meier product limit estimates demonstrate that 24% will be alive disease-free 2 years from transplantation, a result slightly better than that seen in endstage refractory ANL. The actuarial risk of relapse was slightly less in this group than in endstage patients (50% versus 65%). In an effort to determine if it is worthwhile to reinduce a patient with relapsed ANL into a second remission prior to transplantation or if one should simply proceed with transplantation at the time of first relapse, we reviewed our experience in 62 patients with ANL transplanted after first relapse (11). In the 17 patients (group 1) no attempt at remission reinduction was made, while in 20 patients (group 2) attempts at reinduction were unsuccessful, and in 25 patients (group 3) a second remission was achieved. Five of 17 patients (29%) in group 1, 2 of 20 (10%) in group 2, and 5 of 25 (20%) in group 3 are surviving 2-5 years from transplantation. Interestingly, the risk of relapse was significantly less in the group transplanted without attempts at reinduction than in the group transplanted in second CR. These results suggest that transplantation directly after first relapse is superior to waiting until patients have endstage refractory disease and that, except for keeping patients in good clinical condition while logistical problems are being solved (e.g., locating a transplant bed, arranging finances, etc.) there is no obvious advantage to reinducing a patient into second CR prior to transplantation. In most published studies of chemotherapy for relapsed ANL, the percentage of patients who will achieve second CR is 30-57%, but the duration of second CR is short and virtually no relapsed patients can be cured with subsequent chemotherapy (12,13). Thus, for patients with ANL who are not transplanted in first remission, transplantation at the first sign of relapse or during second remission is indicated.

2.4 First remission ANL

The results of combination chemotherapy in the treatment of adult ANL have been reviewed (13-15). Recent reports from several cooperative group trials and large single institution studies indicate that approximately 20% of all adults achieving CR have remained disease-free for 5 years or longer (16-18). In 1979 Thomas et al reported on 19 patients who were transplanted from HLA-identical siblings for ANL in first remission (19). Ten of these 19 patients are still alive disease-free now more than 6 years from transplant (20). Other marrow transplant groups have reported similar results of long-term survival of approximately 50% of patients with ANL transplanted in first remission (21-23). These studies suggest that marrow transplantation results in a greater likelihood of long-term disease-free survival than does continued chemotherapy.

However, retrospective comparisons may be misleading. Marrow transplantation studies may have included only younger, healthier patients and may have excluded those patients who suffered significant medical problems during or after induction therapy and those patients who relapsed after initial induction before transplantation could be carried out. Therefore, in 1977 we began a prospective comparison of marrow transplantation versus continued chemotherapy for adult ANL in which we attempted as much as possible to minimize bias by registering all patients prior to initial induction chemotherapy, by identifying all persons excluded from transplantation, and by selecting a control population of chemotherapy patients excluded from transplantation solely because they lacked an appropriate donor.

From May 1977 to July 1982, 111 consecutive adults age 17-50 with newly diagnosed ANL were treated with a combination of daunorubicin, cytosine arabinoside, 6-thioguanine, vincristine and prednisone. Patients achieving complete remission were offered marrow transplantation if they had an HLA-identical sibling or were treated with continued combination chemotherapy including consolidation therapy and intensification courses. Ninety patients (81%) entered complete remission. Forty-four remission patients had available donors. Eleven of the 44 patients were not transplanted. In one case this reflected a medical decision made by the transplant team; the other 10 patients were all offered transplantation but declined. The remaining 33 remission patients with matched donors were accepted for transplantation and comprise the transplant group of this study. Forty-six patients who achieved CR had no HLA-identical siblings and therefore were treated with continued chemotherapy. Three of these patients, because of significant medical problems which developed during induction therapy, would not have been offered transplantation at any time after remission induction even if a matched donor were available. Thus, 43 patients from the chemotherapy group were used for comparison with the transplant group. The chemotherapy group, the transplant group, and the group of patients who refused transplantation were similar with regard to symptom duration prior to diagnosis, presenting symptoms, white count at diagnosis, and distribution of FAB morphologic types. The mean age of the chemotherapy group was 4 years greater than the transplant group.

Seventeen of the 33 transplant patients (52%) are alive and in remission from 1-1/2 to 7 years from remission induction. Three of the seventeen have significant chronic graft-versus-host disease requiring continued immunosuppressive therapy. Among the 43 chemotherapy patients, 12 (28%) are alive with 10 (23%) in continuous first remission. Kaplan-Meier product limit estimates, including 95% confidence limits, for disease-free survival of the 33 transplant patients and the 43 patients in the chemotherapy group are shown in Figure 2. A Cox regression model was used to examine the impact of the treatment regimen (transplantation versus chemotherapy) on outcome and demonstrated that transplantation was associated with a significant increase in early mortality (defined as death within 6 months of obtaining a CR) ($p < 0.001$) and thereafter transplanted patients had a significantly lower risk of both relapse and death ($p = 0.003$ and 0.002 respectively). This study thus demonstrates that for adults age 17-50 with ANL, marrow transplantation after initial remission induction, although associated with an increased risk of early death, leads to a better chance for long-term disease-free survival. The long-term disease-free survival of 50% of patients seen in this prospective study is very similar to the overall Seattle experience.

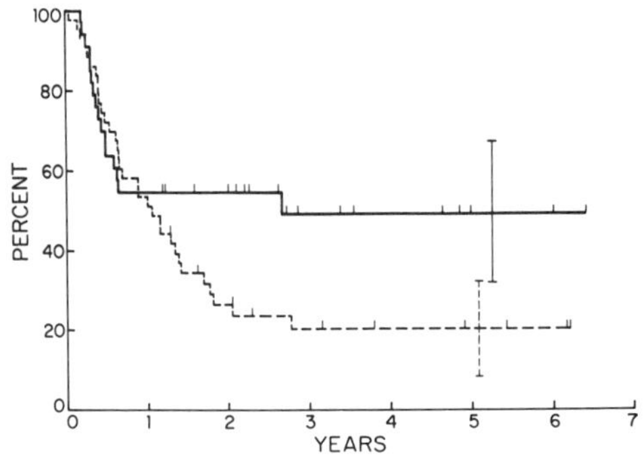

Figure 2. Kaplan-Meier product limit estimates of the probability of disease-free survival (____ transplant group, ---- chemotherapy group). The bars at 5 years are 95% confidence limits. Ticks represent patients alive and in remission.

3. SELECTION OF PATIENTS FOR TRANSPLANTATION IN FIRST REMISSION

A strategy to improve the overall results of the treatment of adults with ANL might be to apply transplantation early in first remission to those patients most likely to benefit from transplantation and to withhold it for certain periods in those patients likely to do well with chemotherapy. At least three general categories of methods may prove useful in this regard.

In the first method, the goal would be to determine if there are common, readily available prognostic indicators which reliably predict the outcome of transplantation or chemotherapy. Patients likely to do well with transplantation and poorly with chemotherapy would be transplanted in first remission while those likely to do well with chemotherapy but poorly with transplantation would have transplantation delayed until first relapse. For example, in our prospective comparative study of transplantation versus chemotherapy, two factors were associated with a significantly shorter duration of CR in the chemotherapy group: FAB morphology of M4, M5 or M6 and a white cell count at diagnosis of over 10,000/mm^3. Neither of these factors influenced the outcome of marrow transplantation. For transplanted patients, only age influenced outcome with patients over age 35 doing worse than younger patients. Thus, the advantage of marrow transplantation is seemingly greatest for younger patients, especially those with high white counts at diagnosis and unfavorable FAB morphology. The advantage is less for older patients, especially those with low white counts at diagnosis and favorable FAB morphology. If prognostic factors are known, Cox regression models can be constructed in which the relative risk of transplantation and chemotherapy can be estimated for different categories of patients. However, the prognostic factors which we have found predictive of remission duration in the chemotherapy group have not been consistently identified in other studies (13). In fact, there are virtually no readily available prognostic indicators which have been universally accepted as being useful in predicting remission duration for patients with ANL. This may reflect the fact that these factors are only weakly associated with remission duration or that they apply only when certain chemotherapeutic programs are used. More work is needed to identify useful predictors of treatment outcome.

A second method of patient selection relies on the results of specific studies of leukemic cell properties. These studies may include cytokinetic studies, *in vitro* sensitivity of leukemic cells to chemotherapeutic agents, assays of the clonogeneic behavior of leukemic cells, cytogenetics, or categorization of leukemic cells by panels of monoclonal antibodies reactive with myeloid differentiation antigens (24-26). Such studies are the subject of other papers in this symposium and will not be reviewed here. But in general, although the results of these assays may reflect differences in remission duration, it remains unclear whether these techniques can reproducibly identify patients who have a high likelihood of cure with chemotherapy. Further, there is as yet no information about how the results of these studies relate to the outcome of marrow transplantation.

A third approach would take advantage of assays designed to attempt to identify impending relapse in ANL patients. These assays include changes in marrow labelling indices (25), premature chromosome condensation (27), antibody detection of residual leukemic cells in the marrow (28), or an increase in circulating immune complexes (29). Theoretically, one could withhold transplantation in all patients until an impending relapse was identified. Unfortunately, these techniques have been studied only in small series and none have been entirely reliable. Further, there is no information about the outcome of transplantation in patients with "impending" relapse.

4. SUMMARY

Marrow transplantation is a form of therapy which offers patients with ANL and a matched sibling a chance of being cured. For patients with refractory disease from the start and those who have relapsed, the chance of cure with transplantation is better than that with chemotherapy. Overall, transplantation in first remission offers the best chance for cure. Attempts are now being made to select appropriate patients for transplantation in first remission. The assumption behind this approach is that it may be possible to select subgroups of patients for whom the chance of cure with transplantation in first remission is less than the chance of cure with the combination of initial chemotherapy and the use of transplantation as salvage therapy if the patient relapses. For such a strategy to be workable, accurate predictors of cure are needed. Further, more information is needed about the outcome of transplantation in first relapse or in second remission, particularly in patients excluded from transplantation in first remission because they were thought to be poor candidates. Finally, information is needed about the outcome of transplantation in patients with "impending" relapse. Transplantation and chemotherapy are not mutually exclusive approaches to the treatment of ANL. The challenge of how best to integrate the two continues.

5. ACKNOWLEDGMENTS

The authors thank the physicians, nurses, ward clerks, secretaries and technologists of the Fred Hutchinson Cancer Research Center and the University of Washington Medical Center for their cooperation in these studies.

This investigation was supported by Grants CA 15704, CA 18029, CA 18221 and CA 30924, awarded by the National Cancer Institute, DHHS. Dr. Thomas is the recipient of Research Career Award AI 02425 from the National Institute of Allergy and Infectious Diseases.

REFERENCES

1. Clift RA, Hansen JA, Thomas ED, Buckner CD, Sanders JE, Mickelson EM, Storb R, Johnson FL, Singer JW, Goodell BW: Marrow transplantation from donors other than HLA-identical siblings. Transplantation 28:235-242, 1979.
2. Thomas ED, Storb R, Clift RA, Fefer A, Johnson FL, Neiman PE, Lerner KG, Glucksberg H, Buckner CD: Bone-marrow transplantation. N. Engl. J. Med. 292:832-843, 895-902, 1975.
3. Buckner CD, Clift RA, Thomas ED, Sanders JE, Stewart PS, Storb R, Sullivan KM, Hackman R: Allogeneic marrow transplantation for acute non-lymphoblastic leukemia in relapse using fractionated total body irradiation. Leuk. Res. 6: 389-394, 1982.
4. Badger C, Buckner CD, Thomas ED, Clift RA, Sanders JE, Stewart PS, Storb R, Sullivan KM, Shulman H, Flournoy N: Allogeneic marrow transplantation for acute leukemia in relapse. Leuk. Res. 6:383-387, 1982.
5. Santos GW, Tutschka PJ, Brookmeyer R, Saral R, Beschorner WE, Bias WB, Braine HG, Burns WH, Elfenbein GJ, Kaizer H, Mellits D, Sensenbrenner LL, Stuart RK, Yeager AM: Marrow transplantation for acute nonlymphocytic leukemia after treatment with busulfan and cyclophosphamide. N. Engl. J. Med. 309:1347-1358, 1983.

6. Glucksberg H, Cheever MA, Farewell VT, Fefer A, Sale GE, Thomas ED: High-dose combination chemotherapy for acute nonlymphoblastic leukemia in adults. Cancer 48:1073-1081, 1981.
7. Preisler H, Anderson K, Rai K, Cuttner J, Yates J: Comparison of survival of patients with acute nonlymphocytic leukemia receiving maintenance chemotherapy or marrow transplantation in 1st remission. ASCO (abstract C691), 177, 1983.
8. Thomas ED, Buckner CD, Banaji M, Clift RA, Fefer A, Flournoy N, Goodell BW, Hickman RO, Lerner KG, Neiman PE, Sale GE, Sanders JE, Singer J, Stevèns M, Storb, R, Weiden PL: One hundred patients with acute leukemia treated by chemotherapy, total body irradiation, and allogeneic marrow transplantation. Blood 49:511-533, 1977.
9. Thomas ED: Marrow transplantation for malignant diseases (Karnofsky Memorial Lecture). J. Clin. Oncol. 1:517-531, 1983.
10. Buckner CD, Clift RA, Thomas ED, Sanders JE, Hackman R, Stewart PS, Storb R, Sullivan KM: Allogeneic marrow transplantation for patients with acute non-lymphoblastic leukemia in second remission. Leuk. Res. 6:395-399, 1982.
11. Appelbaum FR, Clift RA, Buckner CD, Stewart P, Storb R, Sullivan KM, Thomas ED: Allogeneic marrow transplantation for acute nonlymphoblastic leukemia after first relapse. Blood 61:949-953, 1983.
12. Peterson BA, Bloomfield CD: Re-induction of complete remissions in adults with acute non-lymphocytic leukemia. Leuk. Res. 5:81-88, 1981.
13. Foon KA, Gale RP: Controversies in the therapy of acute myelogenous leukemia. Am. J. Med. 72:963-979, 1982.
14. Gale RP: Advances in the treatment of acute myelogenous leukemia. N. Engl. J. Med. 300:1189-1199, 1979.
15. Lister TA, Rohatiner AZS: The treatment of acute myelogenous leukemia in adults. Semin. Hematol. 19:172-192, 1982.
16. Weinstein HJ, Mayer RJ, Rosenthal DS, Coral FS, Camitta BM, Gelber RD: Chemotherapy for acute myelogenous leukemia in children and adults: VAPA update. Blood 62:315-319, 1983.
17. Yates J, Glidewell O, Wiernik P, Cooper MR, Steinberg D, Dosik H, Levy R, Hoagland C, Henry P, Gottlieb A, Cornell C, Berenberg J, Hutchison JL, Raich P, Nissen N, Ellison RR, Frelick R, James GW, Falkson G, Silver RT, Haurani F, Green M, Henderson E, Leone L, Holland JF: Cytosine arabinoside with daunorubicin or adriamycin for therapy of acute myelocytic leukemia: A CALGB study. Blood 60:454-462, 1982.
18. Keating MJ, Smith TL, McCredie KB, Bodey GP, Hersh EM, Gutterman JU, Gehan E, Freireich EJ: A four-year experience with anthracycline, cytosine arabinoside, vincristine and prednisone combination chemotherapy in 325 adults with acute leukemia. Cancer 47:2779-2788, 1981.

19. Thomas ED, Buckner CD, Clift RA, Fefer A, Johnson FL, Neiman PE, Sale GE, Sanders JE, Singer JW, Shulman H, Storb R, Weiden PL: Marrow transplantation for acute non-lymphoblastic leukemia in first remission. N. Engl. J. Med. 301:597-599, 1979.
20. Thomas ED: Marrow transplant for acute nonlymphoblastic leukemia in first remission: A follow-up. (Letter.) N. Engl. J. Med. 308:1539-1540, 1983.
21. Powles RL, Morgenstern G, Clink HM, Hedley D, Bandini G, Lumley H, Watson JG, Lawson D, Spence D, Barrett A, Jameson B, Lawler S, Kay HEM, McElwain TJ: The place of bone-marrow transplantation in acute myelogenous leukemia. Lancet i:1047-1050, 1980.
22. Kersey JH, Ramsay NKC, Kim T, McGlave P, Krivit W, Levitt S, Filipovich A, Woods W, O'Leary M, Coccia P, Nesbit ME: Allogeneic bone marrow transplantation in acute nonlymphocytic leukemia: A pilot study. Blood 60:400-403, 1982.
23. Forman SJ, Spruce WE, Farbstein MJ, Wolf JL, Scott EP, Nademanee AP, Fahey JL, Hecht T, Zaia JA, Krance RA, Findley DO, Blume KG: Bone marrow ablation followed by allogeneic marrow grafting during first complete remission of acute nonlymphocytic leukemia. Blood 61:439-442, 1983.
24. Preisler HD: An integrated approach to the study and treatment of acute myelocytic leukemia. In: Bloomfield CD, ed. Adult Leukemias 1. The Hague: Martinus Nijhoff, 1982, pp. 155-197.
25. Stryckmans P, Debusscher L, Ronge-Collard E, Socquet M, Zittoun R: The labelling index of marrow myeloblasts: A predictive test for relapse of acute non-lymphoblastic leukemia. Leuk. Res. 4:79-87, 1980.
26. McCulloch EA, Curtis JE, Messner HA, Senn JS, Germanson TP: The contribution of blast cell properties to outcome variation in acute myeloblastic leukemia (AML). Blood 59: 601-608, 1982.
27. Hittelman WN, Broussard LC, Dosik G, McCredie KB: Predicting relapse of human leukemia by means of premature chromosome condensation. N. Engl. J. Med. 303:479-484, 1980.
28. Baker MA, Falk JA, Carter WH, Taub RN and the Toronto Leukemia Study Group: Early diagnosis of relapse in acute myeloblastic leukemia: Serologic detection of leukemia-associated antigens in human marrow. N. Engl. J. Med. 301:1353-1357, 1979.
29. Carpentier NA, Fiere DM, Schuh D, Lange GT, Lambert P-H: Circulating immune complexes and the prognosis of acute myeloid leukemia. N. Engl. J. Med. 307:1174-1180, 1982.

13

TREATMENT CHOICES FOR PATIENTS WITH ACUTE NONLYMPHOCYTIC LEUKEMIA IN REMISSION: CHEMOTHERAPY AND BONE MARROW TRANSPLANTATION

Harvey D. Preisler, M.D.

Currently a controversy exists regarding the roles of bone marrow transplantation and chemotherapy in the treatment of acute nonlymphocytic leukemia (ANLL). While each therapeutic approach has dedicated proponents, it is clear that these therapeutic modalities should not be considered as competitors but rather as alternate and complimentary therapies. This paper will attempt to review each approach impartially, and then propose an approach to the treatment of patients with ANLL. The discussion will be limited to patients who enter complete remission at the time of initial diagnosis.

1. CHEMOTHERAPEUTIC APPROACHES

The usual approaches to the treatment of patients who enter remission involve the administration of monthly courses of chemotherapy, i.e., maintenance chemotherapy (1-3). These courses of chemotherapy produce mild degrees of leukopenia and thrombocytopenia (WBC does not fall below 1000 or platelet count below 50,000) and therapy is administered for 3-5 years.

The remission duration curves of the different maintenance regimens are essentially identical in shape and similar at all time points with median durations of remission of 8-14 months with approximately 20% of patients alive and well at 5 years (1-3). Inspection of the details of these regimens suggests for conventional maintenance therapy, the exact agents administered makes little difference. Several reports have suggested that the 20% long term survivors may be cured (4). To define the therapeutic efficacy of conventional maintenance chemotherapy, we reviewed the data for all CALBG patients with ANLL who entered complete remission between 1974 and 1979 (5). Figure 1 provides the remission duration curve for this study. Inspection of the curve demonstrates that this relapse curve has two components, an early high rate of relapse and a lower rate of relapse extending for at least 7 years. Clearly, at no point in time is the patient free of risk of recurrent leukemia. Additionally, it should be noted that the slope of the late component of the relapse curve is so shallow that if a smaller number of patients were followed one might not be able to distinguish between a shallow slope and a "plateau".

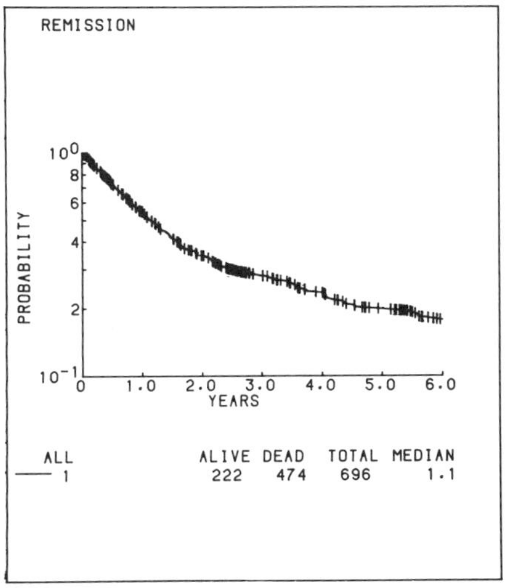

Figure 1. Remission duration curve for 696 patients treated on CALGB protocols who achieved a CR between 1974 and 1979. All patients received monthly courses of maintenance chemotherapy.

The fact that with conventional maintenance therapy leukemic relapse begins as soon as the patient enters remission together with the modest median durations achieved and the fact that the majority of patients relapse has led some investigators to administer consolidation/maintenance regimens which are more aggressive than conventional maintenance therapy. One approach has utilized 14 months of therapy (6) while another has utilized only 4 courses of aggressive consolidation therapy (7). The latter program, initiated at Roswell Park Memorial Institute together with colleagues at the Ontario Cancer Foundation in Hamilton Ontario (Dr. G. Browman), was joined by colleagues at the University of Chicago (Dr. Larson) and at Tufts University (Dr. Miller). Figure 2a provides the schema for the protocol while Figure 2b presents an initial analysis of this study with the data superimposed on the CALGB data. It can be seen that for the aggressively treated patients relapses do not begin as soon as patients enter remission, rather they are delayed until the end of consolidation chemotherapy. Once they begin, however, their curve parallels that of the CALGB data suggesting that intensive consolidation did not substantially alter the natural history of the disease. This appears to be the case for at least the first several years. Longer follow-up time will be necessary to define the long term efficacy of this program.

The data presented in Figure 2b represents all patients who entered remission, whether or not they actually received the prescribed courses of therapy. Figure 3 divides the patients into two groups: those that received the therapy as prescribed and those who did not receive the therapy for reasons other than leukemic relapse or persistent cytopenia. These data demonstrate that the efficacy of intensive consolidation chemotherapy may be greater than would be suspected if the conventional method of analysis is employed, i.e., analyzing all patients together whether or not the patients actually received the therapy. When conventional maintenance type therapy is administered protocol violations do not appear to be of consequence, possibly because the therapy itself is not very effective. Further follow-up is necessary before the long term effects of aggressive consolidation chemotherapy are known.

2. BONE MARROW TRANSPLANTATION IN 1ST REMISSION

The demonstration that bone marrow allografts were potentially curative for patients with relapsed leukemia led to its use in the treatment of patients with minimal residual disease, patients in first hematologic remission (8-10). The reports suggest that this approach to therapy might be curative. In evaluating the efficacy of this approach one must recognize the age dependance of this therapy and pay careful attention to the age distribution of reported studies since those which are comprised primarily of children will demonstrate a therapeutic efficacy which will be irrelevant for the majority of patients with ANLL since the median age at diagnosis of ANLL is 51 years and at remission is 41 years (5).

(A)

(B)

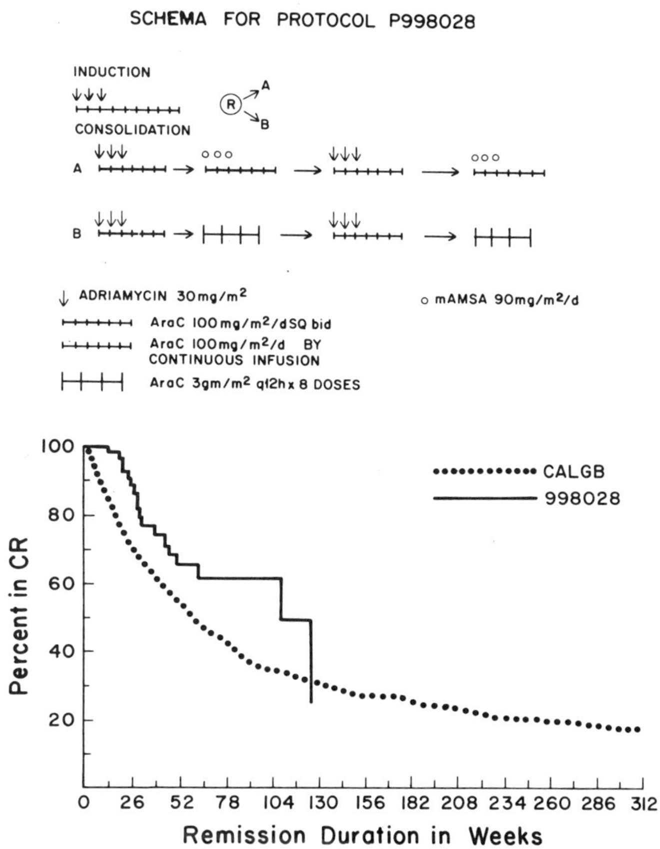

Figure 2. Aggressive Consolidation Chemotherapy a) schema for protocol 998028 b) overall remission durations: comparison of all patients registered on PPC 998028 vs. CALGB study.

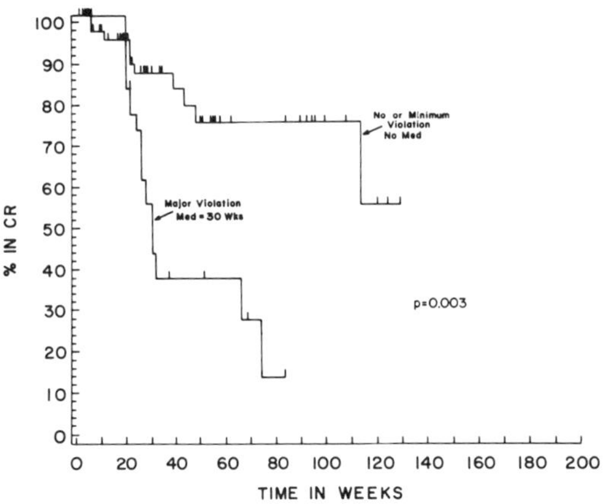

Figure 3. Remission duration curves for patients treated on protocol 998028 divided on the basis of whether or not they were treated according to the protocol.
Major violations - patients in whom 2 of the 4 consolidation courses were either not given at all, were given after a delay of >2 weeks after the time that treatment was supposed to have been started, or patients in whom <80% of the total projected drug dose was administered in 2 of the 4 courses.

Age dependent analysis of the data demonstrates that for patients <20 years of age transplantation provides long term leukemia control in 70% of patients (11). A similar degree of leukemic growth control is produced in patients over 30 years of age but the majority of patients in this age range succumb to the complications of the transplant procedure (11). The median duration of survival is only 6 months with 60-70% of patients >30 y.o. expiring by the end of the first year after transplantation.

3. COMMENTS ON THE SELECTION OF THERAPY FOR PATIENTS WITH ANLL IN REMISSION

The long term results of conventional maintenance therapy has been well defined. The median duration of remission is in the range of 1 year with 18% of patients still in remission at 6 years. Through at least 7 years of remission, there is no evidence for the existence of a plateau phase during which the patient is free of the risk of leukemic recurrence. The therapeutic efficacy of intensive consolidation chemotherapy has not as yet been defined. It seems clear that at the very least such intensive therapy reduces the rate of early relapse and may increase the median duration of remission. Additionally, the data presented here demonstrates that 4 courses of consolidation therapy is at least as good as 5 years of maintenance therapy. Unfortunately, once relapses begin, the shape of the relapse curve appears to be identical to that of the conventional maintenance curves. The long term effects of this therapy will not be known for several more years and the effects of such therapy when administered as prescribed by the protocol are also as yet undefined.

When these data are compared to that of bone marrow allografts several tentative conclusions can be drawn. Bone marrow transplantation in remission is superior to conventional maintenance therapy for patients <25 years of age through at least the first 5 years. It should be remembered, however, that the long term complications of bone marrow transplantation have not been defined and that the existence of a true relapse - free state has been brought into question by the recent occurrence of a relapse 6 years after transplantation (12).

For patients $\geq$ 30 years of age the mortality rate associated with bone marrow transplantation during the first year of remission is substantially higher than that associated with conventional maintenance therapy (13). With the 60-70% transplant mortality rate during the first year and the absence of a documented plateau phase, it would seem that chemotherapy is the current treatment of choice patients $\geq$ 30 years of age and that bone marrow transplantation should be reserved for these patients when their illness relapses. The issues regarding both transplantation and chemotherapy are discussed in detail in an editorial comment that accompanied as recent updating of both chemotherapy and bone marrow transplantation as therapeutic modalities in the treatment of acute leukemia (14).

ACKNOWLEDGEMENT

This work was supported by National Cancer Institute Grant CA-5834.

REFERENCES

1. Rai KR, Glidewell O, Holland JF et al: Treatment of acute myelocytic leukemia: A study by cancer and leukemia group B. Blood 58:1203-1212, 1981.
2. Rees JKL, Sandler RM, Challener J et al: Treatment of acute myeloid leukemia with a triple cytotoxic regimen (DAT). British Journal of Cancer 36:770-776, 1977.
3. Preisler HD, Bjornsson S, Henderson ES et al: Treatment of acute nonlymphocytic leukemia: Use of anthracycline - cytosine arabinoside induction therapy and a comparison of two maintenence regimens. Blood 53:455-464, 1979.
4. Keating MJ: Factors influencing disease free interval after achieving complete remission in acute leukemia. In: Minimal Residual Disease in Acute Leukemia. Lowenberg B, Hagenbeek A (eds) Martinus Nijhoff, Boston, The Hague, Dordrecht, Lancaster, 1984, pp. 149-164.
5. Preisler H, Anderson K, Rai K et al: Comparison of survival of patients with acute nonlymphocytic leukemia receiving maintenance chemotherapy or marrow transplantation in 1st remission. Abstracts of ASCO 5/22-5/24, 1983.
6. Weinstein JD, Mayer RJ, Rosenthal DS et al: Treatment of acute myelogenous leukemia in children and adults. New Eng. J. Medicine 303:473-478, 1981.
7. Preisler HD, Brecher M, Browman G et al: The treatment of acute myelocytic leukemia in patients 30 years of age and younger. Am. J. Hem. 13:189-198, 1982.
8. Thomas, ED, Buckner CD, Clift RA et al: Marrow transplantation for acute nonlymphoblastic leukemia in first remission. New Eng. J. Med. 301:597-599, 1979.
9. Powles RL, Morgenstern G, Clink HM et al: The place of bone marrow transplantation in acute myelogenous leukemia. Lancet 1:1047-1050, 1980.
10. Forman SJ, Blume KG: Bone marrow transplantation for leukemia. In: Hematology 1: Leukemias. Goldman JM, Preisler HG (eds) Butterworths, London, Boston, 1984, pp. 322-329.
11. Thomas ED, Clift RA, Buckner CD: Marrow transplantation for patients with acute nonlymphoblastic leukemia who achieve a first remission. Cancer Treat. Rep. 66:1463-1466, 1982.
12. Applebaum F: Personal communication, 1984.

13. Preisler HD: Bone marrow transplantation for adults over 30 years of age with acute nonlymphocytic leukemia. In: Current Drugs and Methods of Cancer Treatment. Chap 24, pp. 127-128, 1983.
14. Preisler HD: Therapy for patients with acute myelocytic leukemia who enter remission: Bone marrow transplantation or chemotherapy? Cancer Treat. Rep. 66:1467-1473, 1982.

14

AUTOLOGOUS BONE MARROW TRANSPLANTATION IN ACUTE LEUKEMIA

Voravit Ratanatharathorn, Chatchada Karanes, Fr. Joe Mahoney, Frederick R. Appelbaum

With the advent of effective induction chemotherapy for acute leukemia and the development of successful cryopreservation techniques, the clinical study of ABMT as a treatment modality for acute leukemia has now become possible (1). ABMT for the treatment of acute leukemia has its own unique problems and advantages, some of which are summarized in Table 1.

TABLE 1

Autologous BMT: Advantages and Disadvantages

Advantages

1) No donor required
2) No immunologic barrier, i.e., graft rejection or graft versus host disease
3) Lesser degree of post-transplant immune deficiency

Disadvantages

1) Not an option for patients who failed to achieve a complete remission
2) Possible contamination of clonogenic leukemic cells
3) Relative deficiency of hematopoietic stem cells due to previous exposure to cytotoxic drugs
4) Cell loss during marrow preparation, freezing and thawing process

In this chapter we will review the current status of ABMT with emphasis on the role of bone marrow purging, the question of the optimal cytoreductive regimen, and the future direction of this treatment modality.

1. BONE MARROW PURGING - IS IT NECESSARY?

The clonogenicity demonstrated in experimental leukemia in mice has had a major impact upon the design of therapeutic strategies for humans. This subject is reviewed by Valeriote in Chapter 2. The concept of clonogenicity suggests that if cure is to be achieved, every clonogenic leukemic cell must be killed (2). An obvious correlate is that re-infusion of any tumor cells along with cryopreserved autologous marrow following marrow-ablative therapy will inevitably lead to relapse. The actual contribution to tumor relapse by tumor re-infusion in humans is unknown and, in fact, there have been some surprising outcomes which raise real questions. For example, in a study in which 14 patients with relapsed Burkitt's lymphoma were treated with high-dose chemotherapy (BACT) followed by ABMT using remission marrow, three patients continue to survive free of disease, all more than 5 years from transplant (3). The longest survivor is a patient who had marrow involvement at the time of diagnosis, was treated to complete remission at which time his marrow was stored, and eventually relapsed in his marrow prior to ABMT. Despite the fact that his marrow had been previously involved, re-infusion of remission marrow did not lead to relapse (4). Recently, another study has shown that Burkitt's lymphoma cell lines can be established even in human marrow that is microscopically normal (5). These two studies serve to highlight a major clinical problem in ABMT--it is impossible to state with certainty whether a bone marrow is or is not contaminated, or what size of tumor inoculum is necessary to maintain an expanding clone in order to result in relapse. Thus, while bone marrow purging (elimination of clonogenic leukemic cells) is often considered theoretically essential for long-term remission or cure, this issue remains unsettled.

Nonetheless, based on the concept that tumor contamination of marrow may lead to relapse, methods to remove tumor cells from marrow have been developed.

1.1 Marrow fractionation by discontinuous albumin gradients

This technique has been shown to reduce contaminated leukemic cells by 50-90% (6). A subsequent clinical study of 21 evaluable patients, 10 of whom received fractionated autologous marrow rescue, showed no difference in leukemic relapse between the two groups (7).

1.2 In vitro bone marrow treatment with cytotoxic agents

A few cytotoxic agents have been shown to exert a differential lethal effect on normal vs. leukemic progenitor cells *in vitro*, e.g., anthracyclines (8), VP-16-213, 4-Hydroperoxycyclophosphamide (4-HC) (10,11). Among these agents, 4-HC has been the most extensively studied. Transplantation in rats with a mixture of BN derived leukemic and normal marrow cell (10^6 and 64×10^6) demonstrated that a majority became long-term survivors when given marrow incubated with 4-HC at a concentration of 60 nmole/ml, while all the animals died as a result of leukemic relapse when transplanted with untreated bone marrow (11). *In vitro* dose-ranging studies in humans are now underway. Combinations of agents may enhance the effectiveness of this technique, e.g. 4-HC and VP-16-213 (12).

1.3 In vitro bone marrow treatment with antibody

The most intensively investigated approach to cleaning up marrow has focused on the use of antibodies reactive primarily with antigens found on leukemic cells. Although these antigens may be found on some normal cells, the normal cells are either non-essential or do not bear the antigen that allows extensive lysis. Therefore with the addition of a complement to mediate cytolysis or using antibody-toxin conjugate, the action is highly selective against leukemic cells, resulting in sufficient sparing of hematopoietic stem cells to allow engraftment. In animal models, it has been estimated that a 2 or more log reduction of tumor cells can be achieved despite a 500-fold excess of normal marrow cells. Transplantation using antibody-treated marrow is now undergoing initial trials in man (13,14,15).

To evaluate the clinical impact of bone marrow purging in ABMT, one would either have to carry out a controlled randomized trial comparing the results of purged vs non-purged marrow or to compare the results of purged marrow to the results obtained in syngeneic bone marrow transplantation (SBMT) using identical preparative regimens, since syngeneic marrow is not contaminated by leukemic cells. A randomized trial of purged vs. non-purged marrow would require a large number of patients carefully stratified to each arm to detect impact of purging since, based on allogeneic and syngeneic studies, 70% or more of the patients will relapse due to residual tumor in the patients following the preparative regimens. Thus, if purging techniques worked perfectly, no better tha 20-30% cure rate would be expected in most clinical situations. The outcome using unpurged marrow is unknown but may be as high as 10-15% (see below). A study attempting to identify a difference between 10 and 20% would obviously be quite difficult. Furthermore, a comparison of ABMT results to SBMT results may be misleading in that healthy marrow and lymphocytes could conceivably impart an antileukemic effect not present in autologous marrow. Nonetheless, such a comparison is probably worthwhile since it may yield some insight into the value of marrow purging.

2. AUTOLOGOUS BONE MARROW TRANSPLANTATION OF ANL & ALL IN RELAPSE

From the literature we have summarized the experience of ABMT and SBMT in acute non-lymphocytic (ANL) and lymphocytic leukemias (ALL) in relapse (16-35) (See Tables 2 & 3). For

TABLE 2

Results of Autologous and Syngeneic BMT of ANL in Relapse

Authors (Ref)	# Relapse	# Patients	Regimens	No. CR	Mos. in CR
A) Autologous BMT with Chemotherapy alone					
Hellriegel (16)	1st	1	CY,ADM,MTX 6-TG,VCR	1	3
Gorin (17)	1st	4	TACC	4	3,5,3,32+
Herve (18)	1st	5	TACC	5	13,12,13,6.5,14
Zander (19)	1st 2nd	2 6	m-AMSA m-AMSA	1 0	4
Zander (20)	1st & 2nd	5	CBV	3	2,6,7
Maraninchi (21)	1st 2nd	3 3	L-PAM	3 3	5,6+,16+ 1.5*,2.5,13+
TOTAL		29		20(69%)	
B) Autologous BMT with TBI-base regimens					
Herve (18)	1st	2	CY,TBI	2	5,5
Schaeffer (22)	1st	1	CY,TBI	1	4.8
WSU (23)	2nd	1	CY,TBI	1	2.8
Buckner (24)	1st	7	CY,TBI	3	2,3.5,7
Dicke (25)	1st & 2nd	12	PIP,TBI	7	3,7,4,2,5+,5+,8+
Total		21		12(57%)	
C) Syngeneic BMT with TBI-based regimens					
Fefer (26)	1st & 2nd	16	CY,TBI	13(81%)	1.4,1.8,2.7, 3,3.8**,3.9,4.9, 6.4,29+,31.1+, 88.4+,89.7+, 103.3+

Note: *Patients relapsed 1.5 months after BMT, was re-induced into remission with chemotherapy and subsequently received another course of high-dose L-PAM and ABMT.

**Patient died in CR from interstitial pneumonitis.

TABLE 3

Results of Autologous and Syngeneic BMT of ALL in Relapse

Authors (Ref)	Purged BM	# Relapse	# Pts.	Regimens	# CR	Mos. in CR
A) Autologous BMT with Chemotherapy Alone						
Herve (27)	None	2nd	1	TACC	0	0
WSU (23)	None	4th	1	BACT	1	6
Zander (19)	None	1st-3rd	3	m-AMSA	0	0
Zander (20)	NS	NS	12	CBV	4	1,2,6,7
TOTAL			17		5(29%)	
B) Autologous BMT with TBI-based Regimens						
Dicke (25)	5 None	2nd-4th	7	PIP,TBI	3	2,2.5,14
Netzel (28)	Het	NS	2	BCNU,CY Ara-C,TBI	2	1+,6
TOTAL			9		5(56%)	
C) Syngeneic BMT with TBI-based Regimen						
Fefer (26)	NA	2nd-4th	18	CY,TBI	11(61%)	1*,6.7,13.6 3.9,4.3,4, 13.6,16.5, 104.2+,74.4+ 70.7+

Note: *Patient died from hepatitis in CR

patients with ANL transplanted in relapse, the CR rate for SBMT (81%) appears to be higher than ABMT (64%). For those who achieved a complete remission following transplantation, product-limit analysis for disease-free survival (DFS) for chemotherapy alone + ABMT (20 patients), TBI-based regimen + ABMT (12 patients) and TBI-based regimen + SBMT (13 patients) yields a median DFS of 6.5, 5.0, and 4.9 months respectively ($p = 0.48$ Mantel-Cox). However, of the 13 patients who achieved a complete remission in the SBMT group, 5 survive free of disease for over two years (Figure 1).

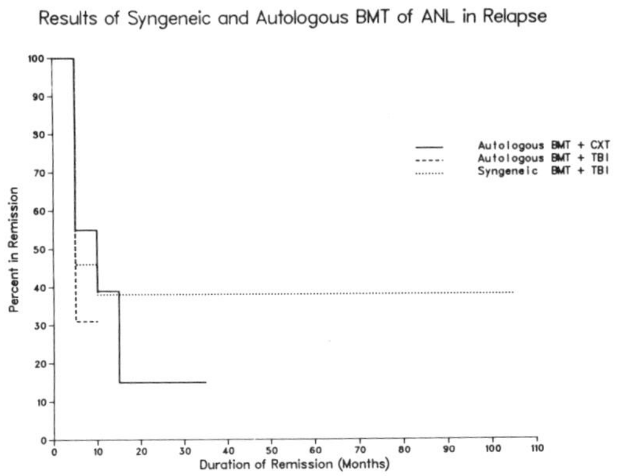

Figure 1. Relapse-free survival of patients with ANL transplanted in relapse.

A similar analysis of the DFS was performed in ALL transplanted in relapse, with a median DFS of: 6 months for chemotherapy alone + ABMT (5 patients), 6 months for TBI-based regimen + ABMT (5 patients) and 13.6 months for TBI-based regimens + SBMT (11 patients) (p = 0.06 Mantel-Cox). In these three groups of patients with ALL, the only long-term survivors were observed in the SBMT group (Figure 2). Given the limitation of

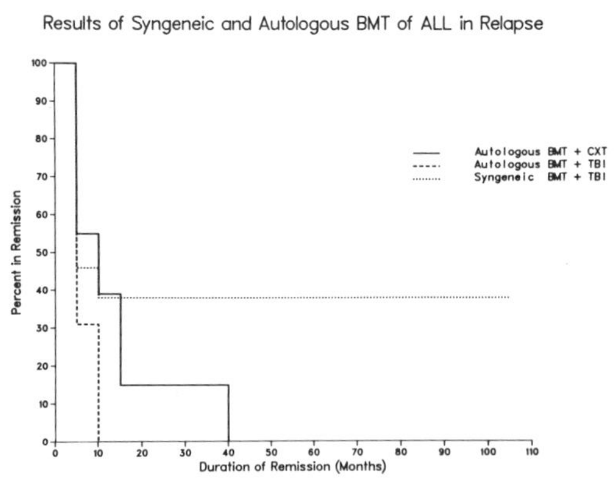

Figure 2. Relapse-free survival of patients with ALL transplanted in relapse.

the small number and shorter follow-up of ABMT patients and the possibility of differences in the patient groups, the results argue for the superiority of SBMT in achieving long term remission and suggest the importance of possible contamination of clonogenic leukemic cells in the transplanted bone marrow. But these results are in no way definitive.

3. AUTOLOGOUS BONE MARROW TRANSPLANTATION OF ANL & ALL IN REMISSION

Because of the lack of detailed report on survival on each individual patient autografted for ANL in remission, comparative analysis can not be made. DFS lasting longer than 20 months has been reported in ANL both for chemotherapy alone and TBI-based regimens (Table 4). With the exception of a small series of 8 patients reported by Herve et al (27) in which the marrows were purged with 4-HC, all the other series employed unpurged marrow (23,24,29,30,31). The significance of marrow purging can not be assessed because of the small number of patients and the difference in cytoreductive regimens (chemotherapy alone vs. TBI).

The presence of common acute lymphoblastic leukemia antigen (CALLA) in 80% of patients with non-T ALL makes *in vitro* marrow purging with J5 monoclonal antibody an ideal model for ABMT. It has been demonstrated that selective depletion of more than 99% of CALLA+ lymphoblasts can be achieved even in the presence of 100-fold normal human marrow cells, thus allowing for subsequent clinical trial. As reported by Ritz (35), 14 patients have been transplanted with J5-treated autologous bone marrow. These patients were transplanted in remission following reinduction chemotherapy, with bone marrow harvested during a second or later remission. Of these, six patients remained in a continuous unmaintained remission at the time of the report, with 4 relapses and 4 deaths within the first three months post-transplant. Two of the 6 disease-free survivors have now been followed for more than 2 years. The result of this series was compared to another group of patients who received allogeneic bone marrow tranplantation from MHC-matched siblings. A relapse rate of 50% was seen in both groups with no difference in survival (35). Another encouraging study was reported by Ramsay et al (34), in which a cocktail of monoclonal antibodies was used for *in vitro* marrow purging.

TABLE 4

Results of Autologous BMT of ANL in Remission

Authors (Ref)	Purged BM	# Relapse	# Pts.	Regimens	ED	# CR	Mos. in CR
A) Chemotherapy alone							
Fay (29)	None	1st	1	BACT	0	1	2
Herve (27)	4-HC	1st	7	TACC	3	0	4+,5+,20+, 20+
		2nd	1		0	1	5
Dicke (30)	None	1st-2nd	6	CBV	0	3	12+ in one other NS
B) TBI-based regimens							
Lowenberg (31)	None	1st	2	CY,TBI	0	NS	4,12+
WSU (23)	None	2nd	3	CY,TBI	1	1	3+
Buckner (24)	None	NS	13	CY,TBI	NS	4	4.5+ - 37+ (4 pts) Two <4 mos

Note: In the series reported by Buckner et al, four patients received post-transplant treatment with human leukocyte interferon (Cantell) and the remaining nine patients received methotrexate with the schedule employed in allograft.

Using discontinuous albumin gradient fractionation, the group at MD Anderson reported their experience of ABMT in 14 patients with ALL in first remission who received 1 or 2 courses of CVB for cytoreduction. There were 3 relapses within 2 months after ABMT and 4 non-leukemic deaths with only 2 patients surviving free of disease at 39+ and 43+ months. The remaining 4 patients relapsed at 4-28 months post-transplant. Seven of the

8 relapses occurred within the first 12 months, which may be a result of inadequate *in vitro* purging of the transplanted bone marrow or a cytoreductive regimen which has not been effective in ablating leukemia in patient. The apparent advantage of transplanting patients in first remission in the MD Anderson series may have been offset by the older age group and heterogeneity of the ALL subtype compared to the results reported by Ramsay et al and Ritz (34,35). While most of the recent studies have used some method of purging, unpurged ABMT has resulted in 3 out of 5 patients surviving at 2.5+, 7+ and 23+ months (at the time when the reports were published) (23,27,32).

If there is a role for marrow purging in ABMT, ALL will be the best model, and perhaps monoclonal antibody will hold the greatest promise. However, the efficacy of using monoclonal antibody remains to be shown in a larger group of controlled clinical trials comparing the remission duration and survival with both purged and unpurged bone marrow.

4. THE QUESTION OF OPTIMAL CYTOREDUCTIVE REGIMENS

Since the majority of patient streated with marrow-ablative regimens have received allogeneic stem cell rescue, several important lessons have been learned from the analysis of this data.

For the past two decades, TBI has been used as an effective means of cytoreduction in bone marrow tranplantation for leukemia. TBI can be delivered as 1,000 rads in a single dose or 1,200 to 1,400 rads in fractionated doses with acceptable extramedullary toxicities. Long-term survival of 5-15% has been reported when high-dose cyclophosphamide and TBI were used followed by allogeneic bone marrow tranplantation in patients with relapsed acute leukemia, and despite advanced disease, a small and yet definitive cure can be achieved with this treatment (34).

Leukemic recurrence is still one of the major reasons of treatment failure in patients who receive cyclophosphamide and TBI followed by allogeneic bone marrow tranplantation, regardless of the status of leukemia at the time of transplant. An analysis of allograft in relapse and in first remission, with exclusion of the competing causes of death, estimates a recurrence of leukemia at 58% and 22% (35,36). The reason for higher recurrence rate for transplant in relapse is twofold, a) extensive exposure to various chemotherapeutic agents may select the more resistant clone(s) which subsequently expands resulting in clinical recurrence (37), b) the tumor burden at the time of cytoreduction plays a critical role in determining the responsiveness to treatment (38). To date, further intensification of the cytoreductive regimens has resulted in a decrease in leukemic recurrence but not in overall survival due to prohibitive toxicities (39). However, it seems unlikely that the best TBI-based regimen has yet been developed. Hopefully better methods of delivering TBI or of combining it with other new chemotherapeutic agents will be developed.

Any comparison of the antileukemic activity of high-dose chemotherapy alone and TBI-based regimens in ABMT is limited by the small number of patients in each of the several regimens reported. Of the various cytoreductive regimens used in ABMT for ANL and ALL in relapse (Tables 2 and 3), the result of chemotherapy alone whether as a single agent or combination was not different from the TBI-based regimens. Remission duration lasting longer than 1 year was observed in several patients with relapsed ANL who received TACC and single agent L-PAM. The patients with relapsed ALL did poorly regardless of the cytoreductive regimens used. Although there are inadequate data to compare TBI-based regimens to those using chemotherapy alone. It should be noted that some long-term disease free survivors are present after the use of chemotherapy-only regimens (Tables 4 and 5). The overall result of cytoreduction with chemotherapy alone is encouraging, and should be further explored because of the potential of selecting synergistic combinations of drugs while avoiding overlapping toxicities. In addition, because an immunologic barrier does not exist in ABMT, one can test a variety of chemotherapeutic regimens for the highest antileukemic activity without considering their immunosuppressive effects. However, it must also be stressed that some of the chemotherapy-only regimens are not truly marrow-ablative and can be delivered without autologous marrow support (e.g. TACC, BACT, and probably CBV). While it is true that the use of autologous marrow in this setting may decrease the period of pancytopenia and thus reduce the risk of severe infections or hemorrhagic complications, this benefit must be weighed against the undefined risk of re-infusing clonogenic tumor cells.

TABLE 5

Results of Autologous BMT of ALL in Remission

Author (Ref)	Purged BM	# CR	# Pts.	Regimen	ED	Mos. in CR
A) Chemotherapy Alone						
WSU (23)	None	4th	1	BACT	0	7+
Dicke (32)	DAGC	1st	14	CBV (x2)	4	1,2,2 (1 Course),4, 10,11,12,28,4*,7*, 11*,16*, 39+,43+ (2 courses)
Dicke (30)	McAb+C	2nd-3rd	4	CBV	1	3,3,5+
B) TBI-based Regimens						
Porcellini (33)	None	1st-3rd	3	CY,TBI	0	3,6,2.5+
Herve (27)	None	2nd	1	CY,TBI	0	23+
Ramsay (34)	BA1,2,3	2nd	12	CY,TBI	NS	1.4,1.9,2.5,3.3,7.5 1*, 5 pts in CCR at 2-16
Ritz (35)	J5 + C'	2nd	14	CY,VM-26 Ara-C,TBI		4 relapse (NS) 4 died in CR 6 in CCR, 2 >2 yrs

Note: *died in complete remission

5. FUTURE DIRECTION OF AUTOLOGOUS BONE MARROW TRANSPLANTATION

The future of ABMT for leukemia will depend upon effective marrow purging and the development of optimal cytoreductive regimens. Any improvement in survival for ABMT patients will depend upon these two critical issues, and therefore they must be addressed in all clinical research protocols. The introduction of various monoclonal antibodies for in vitro treatment and the availability of new chemotherapeutic agents are reasons for optimism. Other issues to be addressed are the selection of candidates for ABMT and the optimal time for bone marrow harvest.

ACKNOWLEDGEMENT

This work was supported in part by the Wayne State University Ben Kasle Trust for Cancer Research.

REFERENCES

1. Deisseroth A, Abrams RA: The role of autologous stem cell reconstitution in intensive therapy for resistant neoplasms. Cancer Treat. Rep. 63:461-471, 1979.
2. Skipper HE, Schabel FM Jr, Wilcox WS: Experimental evaluation of potential anticancer agents. XIII. On the criteria and kinetics associated with "curability" of experimental leukemia. Cancer Chem. Rep. 35:3-111, 1964.
3. Appelbaum FR, Deisseroth AB, Graw RG, Herzig GP, Levine AS, Magrath IT, Pizzo PA, Poplack DG, Ziegler JL: Prolonged complete remission following high dose chemotherapy of Burkitt's lymphoma in relapse. Cancer 41:1059-1063, 1978.
4. Appelbaum FR: Unpublished data.
5. Benjamin D, Magrath IT, Douglass EC, Corash LM: Derivation of lymphoid cell lines from microscopically normal bone marrow in patients with undifferentiated lymphomas: Evidence for occult bone marrow involvement. Blood 61:1017-1019, 1983.
6. Dicke KA, Zander A, Spitzer G, Verma DS, Peters L, Vellekoop L, McCredie KB, Valdivieso M, Lotzova E, McCredie KB: Autologous bone marrow transplantation in relapsed adult acute leukemia and solid tumors. Transplant Proc. 11:212-214, 1979.

7. Dicke KA, Zander A, Spitzer G, Verma DS, Peters L, Vellekoop L, McCredie KB, Hester JP: Autologous bone-marrow transplantation in relapsed adult acute leukemia. Lancet 1:515-517, 1979.
8. Buick RN, Messner HA, Till JE, McCulloch EA: Cytotoxicity of Adriamycin and Daunorubicin for normal and leukemia progenitor cells of man. J. Natl. Cancer Inst. 62:249-255, 1979.
9. Stiff PJ, Wustrow T, Derisi M, Koester A, Lanzotti V, Clarkson B: An in vivo murine model of bone marrow purification of tumor by VP-16-213. Blood 60:173(a), 1982.
10. Korbling M, Hess AD, Tutschka PJ, Kaizer H, Colvin MO, Santos GW: 4-Hydroperoxycyclophosphamide: A model for eliminating residual human tumor cells and T-lymphocytes from the bone marrow graft. Brit. J. Haemat. 52:89-96, 1982.
11. Sharkis SJ, Santos GW, Colvin M: Elimination of acute myelogenous leukemic cells from marrow and tumor suspensions in rat with 4-hydroperoxycyclophosphamide. Blood 55:521-523, 1980.
12. Gulati S, Gandola L, Vega R, Yopp J, Chang TT, Ibrahim S, Siena S, Castro-Malaspina H, Colvin M, Clarkson B: Chemopurification of bone marrow in vitro and its clinical application. Proc. AACR 25:201, 1984.
13. Thierfelder S, Rodt H, Netzel B: Transplantation of syngeneic bone marrow incubated with leucocyte antibodies. Transplantation 23:459-463, 1977.
14. Feeney M, Knapp RC, Greenberger JS, Bast RC Jr.: Elimination of leukemic cells from rat bone marrow using antibody and complement. Cancer Res. 41:3331-3335, 1981.
15. Krolick KA, Uhr JW, Vitetta ES: Selective killing of leukemia cells by antibody-toxin conjugates: Implications for autologous bone marrow transplantation. Nature 295:604-605, 1982.
16. Hellriegel KP, Hirschmann WD, Gauwerky H, Gerecke D, Borberg H, Gross R: Autologous bone marrow transplantation in acute leukemia. In: Cell Separation and Cryobiology, Rainer H (ed), Stuttgart, Schattauer-Verlag, 1978, pp. 335-339.
17. Gorin NC, David R, Stachowiak J, Salmon CH, Petit JC, Parlier Y, Najman A, Duhamel G: High dose chemotherapy and autologous bone marrow transplantation in acute leukemias, malignant lymphomas and solid tumors. Europ. J. Cancer 17:557-568, 1981.
18. Herve P, Rozenbaum A, Plouvier E, Flesh M, Cahn JY, Farradji A, Bergerat JP, Adjizian JC, Pignon B: Autologous bone marrow transplantation in acute myeloid leukemia in relapse or in complete remission. Cancer Treat. Rep. 66: 1983-1984, 1983.
19. Zander A, Vellekoop L, Kicke KA, Keating M, McCredie KB, Legha SS, Spitzer G, Verma DS, Bodey GP: High-dose AMSA and autologous bone marrow transplantation in relapsed acute leukemia. Cancer Treat. Rep. 66:1991-1992, 1982.

20. Zander AR, Dicke KA, Vellekoop L, Verma DS, Kanojia M, Jagannath S, Reading CL, Poynton C, Spitzer G: Autografting in acute leukemia. In: Recent Advances in Bone Marrow Transplantation, Gale RP (ed), Alan R. Liss Inc., NY, 1983, pp. 659-678.
21. Maraninchi D, Abecasis M, Gastaut JA, Sebahoun G, Cahn JY, Herve P, Novakovitch, Carcassonne Y: High-dose melphalan and autologous bone marrow transplantation for relapsed acute leukemia. Cancer Chemother. Pharmacol. 10:109-111, 1983.
22. Schaefer NW: Autologous bone marrow transplantation in acute leukemia. In: Bone Marrow Transplantation in Europe, Touraine JL (ed), Amsterdam, Excerta Medica, 1979, pp. 71-79.
23. Ratanatharathorn V, Karanes C: Unpublished data.
24. Buckner CD, Stewart PS, Bensinger W, Clift RA, Appelbaum FR, Martin P, Sanders J, Fefer A, Lum L, Storb R, Hill R, Thomas ED: Critical issue in autologous bone marrow transplantation for hematologic maligancies. In: Recent Advances in Bone Marrow Transplantation, Gale RP (ed), Alan R. Liss Inc., NY, 1983, pp. 599-613.
25. Dicke KA, Zander A, Spitzer G, Verma DS, Peters L, Vellekoop L, McCredie KB, Hester JP: Autologous bone-marrow transplantation in relapsed adult acute leukemia. Lancet 1:514-517, 1979.
26. Fefer A, Cheever MA, Thomas ED, Appelbaum FR, Buckner CD, Clift RA, Glucksberg H, Greenberg PD, Johnson FL, Kaplan HG, Sanders JE, Storb R, Weiden PL: Bone marrow transplantation for refractory acute leukemia in 34 patients with identical twins. Blood 57:421-430, 1981.
27. Herve P, Philip T, Flech M, Rozenbaum A, Plouvier E, Cahn JY, Noir A, Peters A, Leconte Des Floris R: Intensive cytoreductive regimen and autologous bone marrow transplantation in leukemia. Present status and the future. A review. Eur. J. Cancer Clin. Oncol. 19:1043-1052, 1983.
28. Netzel B, Haas RJ, Rodt H, Kolb HJ, Belohradsky B, Thierfelder S: Antileukemic autologous bone marrow transplantation in childhood acute lymphoblastic leukemia. Transplant Proc. 13:254-256, 1981.
29. Fay JW, Silbermann HR, Moore JO, Noell KT, Hu Hang AT: Autologous marrow transplantation for patients with acute myelogenous leukemia. A preliminary report. Exp. Hematol. 7:302-308, 1979.
30. Dicke KA, Jaganath S, Spitzer G, Poynton C, Zaner A, Vellekoop L, Reading CL, Jehn UW, Tindle S: The role of autologous bone marrow transplantation in various malignancies. Sem. Hemat. 21:109-122, 1984.
31. Lowenberg B, Sizoo W, Sintnicolaas K, Van Bekkum DW, Wagemaker G, Abels J: Experience with autologous bone marrow transplantation in two patients with acute myeloid leukemia in remission. Exp. Hematol. 10:86, 1982.

32. Vellekoop L, Dicke KA, Zander A, Spitzer G, Verma DS, Keating M, McCredie KB: Repeated high dose cyclophosphamide, BCNU, and VP-16-213 and autologous bone marrow transplantation in adult acute lymphocytic leukemia in first remission. Eur. J. Cancer Clin. Oncol. 20:593-599, 1984.
33. Porcellini A, Izzi T, Galimberti M, Moretti L, Polchi P, Lucarelli G: Autologous bone amrrow transplantation in acute leukemia in remission. Exp. Hematol. 10:32, 1982.
34. Ramsay N, LeBien T, Nesbit M, McGlave P, Weisdorf D, Hurd D, Kenyon P, Goldman A, Kim T, Kersey J: Autologous bone marrow transplantation for acute lymphoblastic leukemia following marrow treatment with BA-1, BA-2, BA-3 and rabbit complement. Blood 62(suppl 1):228a, 1983.
35. Ritz J: Use of monoclonal antibody in autologous and allogeneic bone marrow transplantation. Clinics in Haemat. 12:813-832, 1983.
36. Weiden PL, Flournoy N, Thomas ED, Prentice R, Fefer A, Buckner CD, Storb R: Antileukemic effect of graft-versus-host disease in human recipients of allogeneic marrow grafts. N. Engl. J. Med. 300:1068-1073, 1979.
37. Thomas ED, Appelbaum FR, Buckner CD, Clift RA, Deeg HJ, Fefer A, Sanders JE, Singer J, Stewart P, Sullivan KM, Storb R, Witherspoon RP: Marrow transplantation for acute non-lymphocytic leukemia. In: Recent Advances in Bone Marrow Transplantation, Gale RP (ed), Alan R. Liss Inc., NY, 1983, pp. 61-70.
38. Skipper HE, Schabel RM Jr, Lloyd HH: Experiemntal therapeutics and kinetics: Selection and overgrowth of specifically and permanently drug-resistant tumor cells. Sem. Hemat. 15:207-219, 1978.
39. Norton L, Simon R: Tumor size, sensitivity to therapy, and design of treatment schedules. Cancer Treat. Rep. 61:1307-1317, 1977.
40. Gale RP: Approaches to leukemic relapse following bone marrow transplantation. Transplant Proc. 10:167-171, 1978.

List of Abbreviations Used in Tables

ALL : acute lymphocytic leukemia
ANL : acute non-lymphocytic leukemia
BMT : bone marrow transplantation
C' : complement
CCR : continous complete remission
CR : complete remission
DAGC : discontinuous albumin gradient centrifugation
ED : early death
Het : heterologous antibody
McAb : monoclonal antibody
Mos : months
NA : not applicable
NS : not specified
Pts : patients
Ref : reference
ADM : Adriamycin
Ara-C : Cytosine Arabinoside
BCNU : 1,3-bis(2-chloroethyl)-1-nitrosourea
CCNU : 1-(2-chloroethyl)-3-cyclohexyl-1-nitrosourea
CY : Cyclophosphamide
4-HC : 4-hydroperoxycyclophosphamide
L-PAM : 3-[p-[bis(2-chloroethyl)amino]phenyl]-L-alanine
m-AMSA : 4'-(9-acridimylamino)methanesulfon-m-anisidide
MTX : Methotrexate
PIP : Piperazinedione
6-TG : 6-thioguanine
VCR : Vincristine
VP-16-213 : 4'-demethylpipodophyllotoxin 9-(4,6-O-ethylidene--D-glucopyranoside)
BACT : combination of BCNU, cyclophosphamide, Ara-C and 6-thioguanine
CBV : combination of Cyclophosphamide, BCNU and VP-16-213
TACC : combination of CCNU, Ara-C, Cyclophosphamide and 6-thioguanine
TBI : total body irradiation

15

TREATMENT OF LEUKEMIA AND LYMPHOMA WITH BIOLOGICAL RESPONSE MODIFIERS

Kenneth A. Foon, M.D.

1. ABSTRACT

The techniques of genetic engineering, mass cell culture and improved technology in protein and nucleic acid sequencing and synthesis have led to considerable progress over the past 5 years towards the development of specific biological approaches to the treatment of cancer. With this technology, highly purified molecules can be mass produced to be used for cancer therapy. Extensive clinical trials are required to demonstrate that biological response modifiers can provide a survival advantage for patients with cancer, but the preliminary data suggest that these approaches can be useful in inducing responses in patients with certain cancers.

Recombinant and non-recombinant α-interferons have been the most extensively studied biological response modifiers in man. Excellent antitumor activity has been demonstrated against favorable-histology non-Hodgkin's lymphoma, cutaneous T-cell lymphoma and hairy cell leukemia. Less impressive responses for chronic lymphocytic leukemia, unfavorable histology non-Hodgkin's lymphoma and acute leukemia have been reported. Chronic myelogenous leukemia appears to have an intermediate response rate.

Most monoclonal antibodies that react with leukemia- and lymphoma-associated antigens appear to have only transient antitumor effects. The most impressive and durable monoclonal antibody response was reported for a patient with non-Hodgkin's lymphoma treated with an anti-idiotype monoclonal antibody.

Monoclonal antibodies conjugated to radionuclides have been used to image tumors and will eventually be used for therapy as well. In addition, monoclonal antibody treatment of autologous bone marrow to "purge" the bone marrow of malignant cells is being studied at a number of center.

Further studies with biological response modifiers in conjunction with surgery, radiation and chemotherapy should be helpful in definitively establishing biological response modifiers as important modalities for cancer treatment.

2. INTRODUCTION

Progress has been made over the past five years toward the development of specific biological approaches to the treatment of cancer. The techniques of genetic engineering, mass cell culture, and improved techniques in protein and nucleic acid sequencing have made available biologics as highly purified molecules. The most definitive investigations have been carried out with the various interferon (IFN) preparations and it is clear that they are capable of inducing responses primarily in patients with certain types of lymphomas and leukemias. Recent monoclonal antibody data, while interesting, have not yet demonstrated that monoclonal antibodies are effective in the treatment of lymphoma and leukemia. Intensive investigations are currently underway in both of these areas of clinical research.

Historically, there were many attempts to establish immunotherapy as an important modality in the treatment of cancer. There was a considerable body of experimental evidence that alterations of the immune system could be an effective cancer treatment modality in animal models. These data suggested that specific stimulation of the immune response with tumor cells or nonspecific immunologic stimulation with adjuvants such as the Bacillus-Calmette-Guerin (BCG), *Corynebacterium parvum* (*C. parvum*), as well as viruses and bacteria could enhance the existing immune response and delay growth or prevent recurrence of transplanted tumors. However, immunotherapy was not effective in animals bearing palpable tumors. Experimental results suggested that immunologic manipulations or immunotherapy could work only when the tumor cell mass was very small ($<10^6$ cells) (1). This was difficult to translate to the human situation as human malignancies generally had at least two orders of magnitude greater than 10^6 tumor cells at clinical diagnosis. Even in the post-surgical adjuvant setting, the timing of recurrence seems to indicate that larger number of cells were probably present although clinically imperceptible.

Despite the problems suggested in the experimental results with animal tumor models, clinicians began to investigate immunotherapy in the 1970s. Although there were some encouraging nonrandomized preliminary reports, long-term followups were in almost all cases negative. Much of this work is summarized in a recent book on the immunotherapy of cancer (2).

Many of the reasons immunotherapy failed to establish itself as an important therapy for cancer was the lack of purity of the reagents used. Many of the nonspecific approaches involved the use of complex chemicals, bacteria, viruses, and poorly defined extracts, in an attempt to nonspecifically stimulate the immune system. Even in the case of specific immunotherapy, most investigators used cells or cell extracts to try to stimulate the specific immune responses without any molecular definition as to the actual events taking place. Major technological advances over the past five to ten years have given us a strong basis for the new biological therapies. Progress in protein sequencing and synthesis, isolating and purification of biological products, mass cell culture, and the "genetic engineering" of these genes has given us the opportunity to manufacture and test highly purified biologicals and to alter them at the amino acid or nucleotide level to manipulate and optimize their biological activity.

The second major advance was the discovery of the hybridoma technology by Kohler and Milstein (3). The major limitations of the previously popular antisera was the inability to make high-titer specific reagents, reproducible reagents, and produce them in large quantities. With the hybridoma-monoclonal antibody technology, we can now make these immunoglobulin reagents with the same level of molecular purity as cloned gene products and for drugs. Monoclonal antibodies are a powerful tool in the isolation and purification of tumor-associated antigens, lymphokines/cytokines, and other biological molecules which can be used in biological therapy.

Biologicals are products of the mammalian genome. Biological response modifiers are agents and approaches whose mechanisms of action involve the individuals own biological responses. Biologicals and biological response modifiers can act in the following ways: 1) Increase the host antitumor responses through augmentation of effector mechanisms; 2) Increase the host defenses as effectors or mediators of an anti-tumor response; 3) Augment the host responses to modify tumor cells or which might stimulate a greater response by the host for increased tumor-cell sensitivity to an existing response; 4) Decrease the transformation and/or increase differentiation of tumor cells; 5) Increase the ability of the host to tolerate damage by cytotoxic modalities of cancer treatment.

While many of the approaches described above involve the augmentation of host responses, an understanding of the biological properties of the molecules and the immune responses and of the host responses related to growth and maturation will assist in the development of specific molecular entities which have direct actions on both host responses and tumor cells. Thus, one can visualize the development of biological agents with host modifying and direct cytostatic, cytolytic, or maturational effects on tumor cells.

Biological response modifiers can have activity in clinically apparent disease and their testing is not restricted to situations where the tumor mass is imperceptible. The clinical trials designed to test the new biologicals are similar to those used for other modalities of cancer treatment. The primary difference is that one must be sensitive to the need to measure both the pharmacokinetics of the biologics as well as the biological responses affected by these approaches. In clinical trials, the maximum tolerated dose as well as the maximum biological response modifying dose should be established in phase I trials. Both doses may be necessary to test in phase II efficacy trials because a larger quantity of the particular biological response modifier may not necessarily be better therapeutically.

3. RESULTS OF LYMPHOMA/LEUKEMIA INTERFERON TRIALS AT THE NATIONAL CANCER INSTITUTE

IFNs are a family of proteins produced by cells in response to virus, double-stranded ribonucleic acid, antigens, and mitogens. In addition to antiviral activity, the IFNs have profound effects on the immune system. IFNs have direct antiproliferative activity, can alter expression of cell surface antigens, and can influence a number of components of the immune system including B, T, natural killer cells, and macrophages. With respect to the IFNs and cancer therapy, it is still unclear whether the IFNs work primarily by their antiproliferative activity or through alterations of immune responses. It is clear, however, from both the preclinical and clinical studies that IFNs have antitumor activity in a number of tumor systems.

IFNs are currently classified according to various biochemical properties into three groups designated as IFN-α , IFN-β, and IFN-γ. IFN-α and IFN-β (previously grouped together as type I interferons) are acid-stable and are produced primarily by leukocytes and fibroblasts, respectively, in response to viruses or double-stranded ribonucleic acid. Lymphoblastic cells produce a mixture of type I interferon consisting of approximately 90% IFN-α and 10% IFN-β. In contrast, IFN-γ (type II interferon) is an acid-labile IFN produced by T lymphocytes and large granular lymphocytes in response to mitogen or antigen exposure and is ofter referred to as immune IFN.

Most of our studies at the National Cancer Institute have been carried out with IFN-α ; however, we have recently begun a number of phase I IFN-γ trials. Patients entered in our phase I IFN-α trials (4,5) were treated with either a fixed multiple dose of recombinant IFN-α clone A (rIFN-αA from Hoffmann-La Roche, Nutley, NJ) or a single escalating dose of lymphoblastoid IFN-α from human Namalva cells (Burroughs-Wellcome Co., Research Triangle Park, NC). In these phase I trials we determined the maximum tolerated dose of these IFN-αs and observed biological activity, toxicity, and antitumor effects (primarily for lymphomas). Based on the data from our rIFN-αA phase I protocol we designed phase II protocols. In the absence of elucidation of an optimal biological response modifying dose for rIFN-αA, we chose to treat patients in our phase II trials with the maximally tolerated dose of r-IFN-αA with appropriate dose reduction as needed on an individual basis for an acceptable toxicity.

Patients on our phase II lymphoma and leukemia trial were treated with rIFN-αA at a dose of 50 x 10^6 U/m^2 body surface area by intramuscular (i.m.) injection 3 times a week for up to 3 months. Patients were premedicated on the first day of treatment with acetaminophen 600 mg orally every 4 hours, thereafter, acetaminophen was taken as needed. Patients were carefully monitored while on treatment for toxicity by frequent physical examinations and routine laboratory studies. Patients who had unacceptable fatigue (in bed for more than 1/2 day), anorexia (>5% weight loss), intractable nausea and vomiting (requiring i.v. fluids), leukopenia (total leukocyte count <1500/mm^3), or hepatic transaminase elevations (serum aspartate aminotransferase levels >300 IU/ml) were dose-reduced by 50% without interruption of therapy. If there was unacceptable toxicity (defined by the same criteria) at this initial dose reduction, subsequent dose reduction to 10% of the initial dose was instituted.

Patients were monitored for tumor response by frequent measurements of indicator lesions and repeat radiologic studies and photographs as needed. Patient responses were rated according to standard criteria. Patients with objective evidence of tumor regression after three months on the phase II protocol were eligible to continue therapy at the same dosage schedule with monthly reevaluations. Therapy was discontinued immediately if the patient showed objective evidence of progressive disease or if there was no further tumor regression for two successive months.

Ninety-one patients were entered on our phase II lymphoma/leukemia trial. Fifty-one of these patients had non-Hodgkin's lymphoma (NHL), 21 had chronic lymphocytic leukemia (CLL), and 19 had cutaneous T-cell lymphoma (CTCL). Major toxic reactions observed were fever, chills, fatigue, and anorexia. The average duration of therapy at 100% dosage was 2.5 weeks and 6.5 weeks at 50% dose. Fatigue was the most common reason for dose reduction.

Our results indicate significant antitumor activity for rIFN-αA in patients with favorable-histology NHL and CTCL and to a lesser extent CLL. Greater than 50% of the patients with favorable-histology NHL and CTCL responded with either partial or complete responses (Table 1). All responding patients were maintained on rIFN-αA therapy; the median duration of the response is currently in excess of 5 months. The 4 complete responders with favorable-histology NHL were shown to be tumor-free in sites of previous disease by noninvasive studies and biopsies where indicated. The responses in patients with CTCL included reductions of the size of skin plaques and tumors, lymph nodes, and circulating Sezary cells. It was particularly interesting that all of the responding patients had very advanced disease and had failed multiple courses of combination chemotherapy.

These results support previous observations that interferon has activity in patients with favorable-histology NHL (6) and also demonstrates activity in patients with CTCL which was previously not reported. There is less certain activity in patients with CLL and with unfavorable-histology NHL. In the latter case only brief responses were seen in two patients with lymphoblastic lymphoma.

Table 1

Clinical Responses in NCI Phase II rIFN-α A Lymphoma/Leukemia Trial

Disease	Evaluable Patients	Complete Response	Partial Response	Minimal or no Response	Progression
Favorable					
NHL	24	4	10	7	3
Unfavorable					
NHL	11	0	3	2	6
CLL	18	0	2	5	11
CTCL	17	0	9	5	3

IFN-α may have therapeutic value in chronic myelogenous leukemia (7) and is very effective in hairy cell leukemia with 7 of 7 patients responding to a nonrecombinant preparation of IFN-α (3 complete responses) (8).

The activity of IFN-α in acute leukemia has not been extensively studied. In one study, 14 patients with AML who had failed previous therapies received human lymphoblastoid interferon at a dose of 100 x 10^6 U/m^2 daily by intravenous infusion for 7 days (9). While complete remissions were not achieved in any of the 10 patients evaluable for response, a transient decrease in the degree of bone marrow infiltration was observed in 2 patients. Similar results were reported for six other patients with acute leukemia. In another study, five patients with acute lymphoblastic leukemia (ALL), three with AML, and one with blastic transformations of CML received high dose intravenous human leukocyte IFN-α (> 1×10^6 units/kg/day) (11). All of the ALL patients receiving high dose interferon showed definite responses with substantial or complete clearing of leukemia cells from the peripheral blood and bone marrow. One of these patients had previously failed to respond to a 21 day course of lower dose interferon. Two of 3 patients with AML and one patient with blast crisis CML also responded to high dose interferon ($0.5 - 5 \times 10^6$ U/kg/day). Of the 2 patients with AML, both had complete clearing of peripheral blood. One of the patients also had clearing of the bone marrow after one month of therapy. The CML blast crisis patient had more than a 90% reduction in blast cells by the 23rd day. Therapy was discontinued in all of the patients due to a limited supply (11). These encouraging results are clearly unusual and have not been substantiated by other investigators.

4. RESULTS OF LYMPHOMA/LEUKEMIA MONOCLONAL ANTIBODY TRIALS

Monoclonal antibodies are extremely useful in the classification of leukemia and lymphoma (12) and there is considerable interest in the utilization of monoclonal antibodies for treatment as well (13-15). A number of studies utilizing monoclonal antibodies for the treatment of leukemia and lymphoma in animal tumor models (16) and man (17-28) have recently been reported. These studies have emphasized the pharmacokinetics of monoclonal antibody therapy, toxicity, biodistribution, and responses to these murine-derived antibodies (Table 2).

Table 2

Monoclonal Antibody Clinical Trials for Lymphoma and Leukemia

Institution	Disease	Antibody/Class	Specif-icity	No. of Patients	Toxicity	Effect	Ref.
Dana-Farber	B-lymphoma	Ab89/IgG_{2a}	lymphoma	1	renal (transient)	Transient reduction in circulating cells	19
Dana-Farber	cALL	J5/IgG_{2a}	CALLA	4	fever (101-102°F)	Transient reduction in circulating cells	17
Stanford	ATL	L17F12 (anti-Leu-1)/IgG_{2a}	Leu-1	1	renal, hepatic (transient)	Transient reduction in cirulating cells	
Stanford	CTCL	L17F12/IgG_{2a}	Leu-1	6	dyspena, hives, cutaneous pain	Minor remission 5 of 7 patients	14, 24,25
Stanford	T-ALL	L17F12/IgG_{2a} 12E7/IgG_1 4H9/IgG_{2a}	Leu-1 T & B cells T cells	8	sporadic coagulopathy	Transient reduction in circulating cells	14
Stanford	B-lymphoma	4D6/IgG_{2a}	Idiotype	1	none	Complete remission 24+ months	27
U. Calif. San Diego	B-CLL	T101/IgG_{2a}	T65	4	dyspena, hypertension, fever, malaise, urticaria	Transient reduction in ciruclating cells	20
U. Calif. San Diego	CTCL	T101/IgG_{2a}	T65	4	dyspena, fever	Minor remissions	
NCI	B-CLL	T101/IgG_{2a}	T65	13	dyspena, fever (101-102°F), hypotension	Transient reduction in circulating cells	22
NCI	CTCL	T101/IgG_{2a}	T65	8	dyspena, fever (101-102°F)	Minor remission 4 of 8 patients	21
Dartmouth	AML	PM/81/IgM AML-2-23/IgG_{2b} PMN 29/IgM PMN 6/IgM		3	fever arthralgia, myalgia, back pain	Transient reduction in circulating cells	18

4.1 Antibody therapy for acute lymphoblastic leukemia

Four patients with acute lymphoblastic leukemia were treated with escalating doses of the J5 monoclonal antibody, which binds to the common acute lymphoblastic leukemia antigen (CALLA) (17). In this study, patients demonstrated transient reductions in the circulating leukemia cells immediately following therapy with J5 antibody and they demonstrated *in vivo* antibody localization to circulating and bone marrow tumor cells. Antimurine antibody responses were not described; however, resistance to therapy was mediated in part by antigenic modulation of CALLA (loss of antigen from the cell surface membrane) in response to treatment with J5 antibody.

4.2 Monoclonal antibody therapy for acute myelogenous leukemia

A series of IgM monoclonal antibodies recognizing glycolipid determinants on AML cells and an IgG_{2b} antibody recognizing a protein on the surface membrane of AML cells were studied in a serotherapy trial of 3 patients (18). Transient declines in circulating AML cells were reported with evidence for *in vivo* binding to circulating leukemia cells. There was no antigenic modulation demonstrated with any of these antibodies. Human antimurine antibody responses were demonstrated in 1 of 3 patients. Toxicity was limited to mild fevers, back pain, arthralgia, and myalgia.

4.3 Monoclonal antibody therapy for B-cell-derived tumors

The first monoclonal antibody serotherapy trial was reported by Nadler et al. (19). In this study, a patient with B-cell-derived lymphoma was treated with Ab89 in increasing dosages up to 1500 mg infused intravenously over 6 hours. There was a transient reduction in circulating tumor cells as well as a transient drop in creatinine clearance. A number of patients with B-cell-derived CLL have been treated at the University of California, San Diego, and at the National Cancer Institute (20-22). Patients in these studies have been treated with total dosages of the T101 monoclonal antibody ranging from 8 mg to 400 mg (single doses ranging from 1 mg to 140 mg). Transient reductions in circulating leukemia cell counts were described in most of these patients; however, in only 2 patients was there a sustained reduction of 50% of the total circulating leukemia cells throughout the 4 weeks of therapy (22). However, even in those 2 patients, the levels rose to above baseline following the completion of the antibody therapy. There was no responses in lymph nodes or organs in any of these patients. As most of these patients were stage IV by the Rai classification and were hypogammaglobulinemic, it was not surprising that they were unable to mount antimurine antibody responses.

4.4 Cutaneous T-cell lymphoma

A number of groups have treated patients with CTCL with either the T101 monoclonal antibody or the anti-Leu-1 monoclonal antibody, both of which react with the same 65 to 67,000 molecular weight glycoprotein (21,23-25). In these studies, a number of patients demonstrated transient improvements in their cutaneous skin lesions and in some cases, there was shrinkage of enlarged lymph nodes. As these patients were generally immunologically intact, a number of the patients mounted antimurine antibody responses.

4.5 Anti-idiotype antibody therapy for B-cell lymphoma

A more specific approach to the use of monoclonal therapy is the use of anti-idiotype monoclonal antibodies. Immunoglobulin molecules have a unique region in their variable portion termed the idotype. The idiotype for every immunoglobulin molecule is different. As B-cell diseases are clonal diseases, each tumor cell expresses the same immunoglobulin molecule; therefore, the idiotype is identical on every tumor cell. In this unique situation the idiotype is therefore a tumor-specific antigen. A group of investigators from Stanford, led by Dr. Ronald Levy, developed a monoclonal antibody to the idiotypic determinant from a patient with a B-cell lymphoma who had become resistant to cytotoxic drugs and interferon (26). This patient was treated with 8 dosages of anti-idiotype monoclonal antibody intravenously in a dose-escalation fashion and he eventually entered a complete remission which has persisted for over two years. Five additional patients have been treated with less spectacular results (28). Further studies with anti-idiotype antibodies will be necessary before we can determine whether this will be an important therapy. In our own studies at the NCI, we will expect to be treating patients with CLL, nodular lymphoma, and diffuse lymphoma with anti-idiotype monoclonal antibodies in 1984.

4.6 Immunoconjugates

Antibodies conjugated to drugs, toxins and radionuclides can be used for therapy and radioimaging. A considerable body of evidence suggests, at least in animal tumor models, that antibodies covalently linked to certain toxins, such as ricin or diphtheria toxin, have a greater antitumor effect both *in vitro* and *in vivo* than unconjugated free antibody (16,29). A number of centers are currently studying monoclonal antibody conjugates to radionuclides, such as ^{111}indium and ^{131}iodine; to determine whether they can be useful diagnostic tools in man. Over the next few years we anticipate therapy trials in man using toxins, radionuclides and drugs such as doxorubicin (Adriamycin®), covalently linked to monoclonal antibodies in order to determine whether they will have a greater antitumor effect than unconjugated free antibody.

4.7 Clinical toxicity of monoclonal antibodies

One of the major problems witnessed in the NCI clinical trial with T101 was shortness of breath and chest tightness either during or immediately following a 2-hour infusion of T101 at dosages of 50 mg or greater (21,22). This toxicity was eliminated when the infusion of antibody was slowed to 1 to 2 mg/hr. Rare patients have developed hypotension and tachycardia following the infusion of murine monoclonal antibody (20-22). One patient from our study also developed uticaria coincident with hypotension, suggesting that this was an anaphylactic reaction. The hypotension rapidly responded to fluids. Urticaria was a common problem which usually rapidly responded to antihistamines. Fever, chills, flushing, nausea, and vomiting have been reported, but have generally been minor problems. Occasional patients have developed a transient reduction in their creatinine clearance and an elevation of their liver enzymes (19,23) thought to be secondary to immune complexes between monoclonal antibody and circulating antigen. We have also witnessed two cases of serum sickness in patients treated on our antimelanoma monoclonal antibody protocol. In conclusion, murine-derived monoclonal antibodies can be safely infused; however, side effects can be expected but are usually mild.

4.8 Use of monoclonal antibodies in autologous bone marrow transplantation

Another attractive approach to the use of monoclonal antibodies is to "clean up" autologous bone marrow prior to bone marrow transplantation. Patients with acute lymphoblastic leukemia have had bone marrow removed and treated with the J5 monoclonal antibody (29). Following bone marrow removal, treatment and storage, patients were treated with high-dose chemotherapy and radiation therapy and then "rescued" with their J5 antibody-treated autologous bone marrow. A similar approach to therapy has been described using the B1 monoclonal antibody to cleanup autologous bone marrow from patients with non-Hodgkin's lymphoma (30). The results of these trials are preliminary, but have clearly demonstrated that antibody-treated autologous bone marrow is capable of restoring hematopoiesis. Long-term results demonstrating disease-free survival will be necessary before firm conclusions regarding the efficacy of this therapy can be drawn.

4.9 Conclusion

The use of monoclonal antibody and antibody immunconjugates in the treatment of radioimaging of cancer is in its infancy. While such work needs to be done to clarify many of the issues surrounding the use of monoclonal antibodies, it has been clearly demonstrated in both animal tumor models and man that antibody alone and antibody conjugates have a therapeutic effect (16,31). The potential for monoclonal antibodies in cancer therapy is enormous given the specificity that is inherent to the antibody-antigen reaction. We are cautiously optimistic in exploring this exciting new approach to cancer therapy.

ACKNOWLEDGMENTS

I would like to thank Hoffmann-La Roche, Inc. for supplying the rIFN αA and Hybritech, Inc. for the T101 used in the studies described in this manuscript. I am indebted to the staff of the Clinical Investigations and Monoclonal Antibody Sections of the Biological Response Modifiers Program as well as Dr. Paul Bunn of the Navy Oncology Branch and Dr. Dan Longo of the Medicine Branch of the Clinical Oncology Program for their invaluable assistance in carrying out some of the studies described in this manuscript.

This project has been funded at least in part with Federal funds from the Department of Health and Human Services, under contract number NO1-CO-23910 with Program Resources, Inc. The contents of this publication do not necessarily reflect the views or policies of the Department of Health and Human Services nor does mention of trade names, commercial products, or organizations imply endorsement by the U.S. Government.

REFERENCES

1. Oldham RK, Smalley RV: Immunotherapy: The old and the new. J. Biol. Resp. Modif. 2:137, 1983.
2. Terry WD, Rosenberg A: Immunotherapy of human cancer. New York, Excerpta Medica, 1982.
3. Kohler G, Milstein C: Continuous cultures of fused cells secreting antibody of predefined specificity. Nature 256: 495-497, 1975.
4. Sherwin SA, Knost JA, Fein S et al: A multiple dose phase I trial of recombinant leukocyte A interferon in cancer patients. JAMA 248:2461-2466, 1982.
5. Knost JA, Sherwin SA, Abrams PG et al: The treatment of cancer patients with human lymphoblastoid interferon: A comparison of two routes of administration. Cancer Immunol. Immunother. 15:144-148, 1983.

6. Louie AC, Gallagher JG, Sikora K, Levy R, Rosenberg SA, Merigan TC: Follow-up observations on the effect of human leukocyte interferon in non-Hodgkin's lymphoma. Blood 58:712-718, 1981.
7. Talpaz M, Mavligit G, Keating M, Walters RS, Gutterman JU: Human leukocyte interferon to control thrombocytosis in chronic myelogenous leukemia. Ann. Intern. Med. 99:789-792, 1983.
8. Quesada JR, Reuben J, Manning JT, Hersh EM, Gutterman JU: Alpha interferon for induction of remission in hairy cell leukemia. N. Engl. J. Med. 310:15-19, 1984.
9. Rohatiner AZS, Balkwill FR, Malpas JS, Lister TA: Experience with human lymphoblastoid interferon and acute myelogenous leukemia (AML). Cancer Chemother. Pharmacol. 11: 56-58, 1983.
10. Rohatiner AZS, Balkwill FR, Griffin DB, Malpas JS, Lister TA: Phase I study of human lymphoblastoid interferon administered by continuous intravenous infusion. Cancer Chemother. Pharmacol. 9:97-102, 1982.
11. Hill NO, Pardue A, Kahn A, Aleman C, Dorn G, Hill JM: Phase I human leukocyte interferon trials in cancer and leukemia. J. Clin. Hematol. Oncol. 11:23-35, 1981.
12. Foon KA, Schroff RW, Gale RP: Cell surface markers on leukemia lymphoma cells: Recent advances. Blood 60:1-19, 1982.
13. Ritz J, Schlossman SF: Utilization of monoclonal antibodies in the treatment of leukemia and lymphoma. Blood 59:1-11, 1982.
14. Levy R, Miller RA: Tumor therapy with monoclonal antibodies. Fed. Proc. 42:2650-2756, 1983.
15. Oldham RK: Monoclonal antibodies in cancer therapy. J. Clin. Oncol. 1:582-590, 1983.
16. Foon KA, Bernhard MI, Oldham RK: Monoclonal antibody therapy: Assessment by animal tumor models. J. Biol. Resp. Modif. 1:277-304, 1982.
17. Ritz J, Pesando JM, Sallan SE, Clavell LA, Notis-McConarty J, Rosenthal P, Scholossman SF: Serotherapy of acute lymphoblastic leukemia with monoclonal antibody. Blood 58: 141-152, 1981.
18. Ball ED, Bernier GM, Cornwell GG, McIntyre OR, O'Donnell JF, Fanger MW: Monoclonal antibodies to myeloid differentiation antigens: <u>In vivo</u> studies of three patients with acute myelogenous leukemia. Blood 62:1203-1210, 1983.
19. Nadler LM, Stashenko P, Hardy R, Kaplan WD, Button LM, Kufe EW, Antman KH, Schlossman SF: Serotherapy of a patient with a monoclonal antibody directed against a human lymphoma-associated antigen. Cancer Res. 40:3147-3154, 1980.
20. Dillman RO, Shawler DL, Sobel RE, Collins HA, Beauregard JC, Wormsley ST, Royston I: Murine monoclonal antibody therapy in two patients with chronic lymphocytic leukemia. Blood 59:1036-1045, 1982.

21. Foon KA, Schroff RW, Sherwin SA, Oldham RK, Bunn PA, Hsu S-M: Monoclonal antibody therapy of chronic lymphocytic leukemia and T cell lymphoma: Preliminary observations. In: Monoclonal Antibodies and Cancer, Boss BD, Langman RE, Towbridge IS, Dulbecco R (eds.), Academic Press, New York, 1983, pp. 39-52.
22. Foon KA, Schroff RW, Bunn PA, Meyer D, Abram PG, Fer MF, Ochs JJ, Bottino GC, Sherwin SA, Herberman RB, Oldham RK: Effects of monoclonal antibody serotherapy in patients with chronic lymphocytic leukemia. Blood 64:1085-1094, 1984.
23. Miller RA, Maloney DG, McKillop J, Levy R: *In vivo* effects of murine hybridoma monoclonal antibody in a patient with T-cell leukemia. Blood 58:78-86, 1981.
24. Miller RA, Levy R: Response of cutaneous T cell lymphoma to therapy of hybridoma monoclonal antibody. Lancet 2: 225-230, 1981.
25. Miller RA, Oseroff AR, Stratte PT, Levy R: Monoclonal antibody therapeutic trials in seven patients with T-cell lymphoma. Blood 62:988-995, 1983.
26. Hatzubai A, Maloney DG, Warnke R, Levy R: Use of a monoclonal anti-idiotype antibody to study the biology of a human B cell lymphoma. J. Immunol. 126:2397-2402, 1981.
27. Miller RA, Maloney DG, Warnke R, Levy R: Treatment of B-cell lymphoma with monoclonal anti-idiotype antibody. New Engl. J. Med. 306:517-522, 1982.
28. Meeker TC, Maloney DG, Thielmans K, Miller RA, Lowder J, Levy R: Anti-idiotype monoclonal antibody therapy of human B lymphocytic malignancy. Blood 62(suppl 1):214, 1983.
29. Bernhard MI, Foon KA, Oeltmann TN, Key ME, Hwang KM, Clarke GC, Christensen WL, Hoyer LC, Hanna MG Jr, Oldham RK: Guinea pig line 10 hepatocarcinoma model: Characterization of monoclonal antibody and *in vivo* effect of unconjugated antibody and antibody conjugated to diptheria toxin A chain. Cancer Res. 43:4420-4428, 1983.
30. Ritz J, Bast RC, Clavell LA, Hercend T, Sallen SE, Lipton JM, Feeney M, Nathan DG, Schlossman SF: Autologous bone marrow transplantation in CALLA-positive acute lymphoblastic leukemia after *in vitro* treatment with J5 monoclonal antibody and complement. Lancet 2:60-63, 1982.
31. Nadler L, Takvorian T, Finberg R, Bast R, Botnick L, Hellman S, Canellos G, Schlossman S: Autologous marrow transplantation for relapsed non-Hodgkin's lymphoma: Anti- B1 monoclonal antibody treated autologous bone marrow. Blood 62(suppl 1):226, 1983.

16

TRANSFUSION THERAPY FOR THE SUPPORT OF LEUKEMIA PATIENTS

Chatchada Karanes and Voravit Ratanatharathorn

Over the past decade, developments in transfusion medicine have contributed to an increased survival for patients with acute leukemia. Current therapeutic strategies using very aggressive induction, consolidation, and intensification chemotherapy and/or bone marrow transplantation result in severe myelosuppression for at least 2-3 weeks. Consequently, all patients require frequent transfusions of packed red cells and platelets until there are signs of bone marrow recovery; granulocyte transfusions may occasionally be indicated.

Advances in blood bank and pheresis technology now enable us to be highly specific in collecting blood components thereby minimizing transfusion reaction and alloimmunization. Indications and types of blood component replacement for these patients will be discussed. We will examine in detail the rationale for granulocyte transfusions since the clinical issues in such therapy are complex.

1. RED BLOOD CELL TRANSFUSION

The use of saline-washed red blood cells is generally recommended for patients requiring long-term blood support. Using the IBM blood processor, it is possible to prepare a transfusion depleted of over 90% of the granulocytes and 99% of the original plasma. In addition, more than 90% of microaggregates (debris consisting of degenerated leukocytes and platelets) are removed together with undesirable products of red blood cell storage and metabolism, i.e., lactic acid, ammonia, potassium citrate and plasticizer. There are four clinical advantages in using washed packed red cells. First, there is less occurence of the two most common forms of transfusion reaction, namely, febrile, non-hemolytic reaction from contaminated leukocytes and urticarial reaction from contaminated plasma. Second, there is decreased alloimmunization to HLA, granulocyte- and platelet-specific antigens. Third, there is a decrease in the incidence of graft-versus-host disease, which may sometimes occur as a result of the transfusion of allogeneic lymphocytes to immunosuppressed patients, even in the absence of allogeneic bone marrow transplantation. Last, there is a decrease in the incidence of transfusion hepatitis (1).

Any evaluation of the need for red blood cell transfusions during a myelosuppressive period should be based not only on the ability of the patient to compensate, but should include symptoms, signs and risks related to the anemia itself. Although there is no general agreement, many investigators feel that a hemoglobin level of 9-10 gm% should be maintained at all times until bone marrow recovery occurs. It is possible that maintaining the hemoglobin at this level may be effective in diverting the flow of pleuripotential stem cells to the granulocytic series, resulting in a shortened granulocytopenic period; however, this contention is not supported by any firm human data (2).

2. GRANULOCYTE TRANSFUSION

2.1 Therapeutic granulocyte transfusion

During a period of marrow aplasia, the incidence of infection does not increase significantly until there are less than 100-200/cu. mm. of circulating granulocytes (3,4). For example, if a granulocyte level of 100/cu. mm. persists for more than 3 weeks, one can anticipate that virtually all patients will become infected. In addition, the presence or absence of a trend toward granulocyte recovery is a critical prognostic factor. Patients showing such a trend by a consistent daily rise of granulocyte count will do well on antibiotic therapy alone, with an expected 90% cure of infection (5-7).

In an animal study, cyclophosphamide-induced granulocytopenic dogs with pseudomonas sepsis were randomly assigned to receive treatment with antibiotics alone versus antibiotics and granulocyte transfusions. Survival analysis showed a significant improvement with granulocyte transfusions of 1.5 - 2.0 x 10^8/kg/transfusion (obtained from continuous flow centrifugation (8)).

Prospective randomized clinical trials published during 1975-1980 were in favor of granulocyte transfusions for infected granulocytopenic patients, although the patient population was heterogeneous in terms of diagnosis, level of granulocytopenia, type of infection, and the methods for procurement of granulocytes. Herzig et al. (9) studied patients with gram-negative sepsis and granulocyte count of $<$ 1,000/cu. mm. Eight out of 12 patients without bone marrow recovery who received granulocyte transfusions survived, while all patients in the control group died of infection. For patients with granulocytopenia lasting less than 10 days, the benefit of granulocyte transfusion has not been demonstrated (9).

These early studies led to widespread use of granulocyte transfusions in granulocytopenic patients despite its limited efficacy. A more recent, larger, randomized trial at UCLA studied 95 patients with a granulocyte count of less than 500/cu. mm. (10). These patients were randomized to receive or not to receive granulocyte transfusions in addition to antimicrobial therapy, with treatment beginning within 24 hours of microbiological or roentgenographic documentation of infection. Analysis of the response rate with respect to both the type of infection and the bone marrow recovery status in these two groups of patients did not favor the routine use of therapeutic granulocyte transfusion (10).

Because of the heterogeneity and small number of patients in these trials, it is difficult to determine what additional factors may influence the impact of granulocyte transfusions. In an attempt to address this complicated issue, Love et al. (11) undertook a retrospective analysis of 67 episodes of gram-negative bacteremia in granulocytopenic cancer patients. Granulocyte transfusions were instituted for patients with a granulocyte count of <1,000/cu. mm. (median = 100/cu. mm.) who responded poorly to 24-48 hours of appropriate antimicrobial therapy. This study identified the importance of organism sensitivity to the initial antibiotic treatment, especially when granulocytopenia is longer than 14 days. No patient responded who had organisms resistant to both antibiotics used as well as absence of marrow recovery. A response rate of 75% was reported for patients in whom the organism was sensitive to both antibiotics, in spite of the absence of bone marrow recovery (11).

The conflicting data discussed above should be interpreted with caution. It would be premature to preclude entirely the use of therapeutic granulocyte transfusion in infected granulocytopenic patients, but clinicians must exercise discretion. Although there is no general consensus, most investigators will institute therapeutic granulocyte transfusion early in the treatment, i.e., within 48 hours after the initiation of appropriate antimicrobial therapy in patients with a granulocyte count <100/cu. mm. who have severe infection (septicemia, pneumonia or extensive soft tissue infection). Once granulocyte transfusion is initiated, it should be continued for at least 4-7 days or until there is evidence of bone marrow recovery, unless there is a rapid resolution of infection with antimicrobial therapy (12).

2.2 Prophylactic granulocyte transfusion

The rationale for prophylactic granulocyte transfusion is based on the well-documented fact that the relative severity of granulocytopenia is an important risk and prognostic factor. It is conceivable that a relatively small number of transfused granulocytes may be ineffective for patients with established infection, but may be adequate to eradicate early foci of infection. Strauss et al. (13) studied the role of prophylactic granulocyte transfusions during remission induction chemotherapy of acute myelogeneous leukemia. One hundred and two uninfected patients were randomized to receive daily granulocyte transfusions with a granulocyte count <500/cu. mm. or to receive standard therapy alone. Although the percentage of infected patients was similar for both groups, granulocyte transfusions decreased the incidence of bacterial septicemia (9% versus 27%). Another study involving bone marrow transplant recipients also showed that prophylactic granulocyte transfusion significantly reduced the incidence of septicemia in the transfused group (14). However, Strauss et al concluded from their experience that prophylactic granulocyte transfusions should not be used since the risk outweighed the benefit, due to a high incidence of transfusion reaction and increased pulmonary infiltrate in the transfused patient which lead to death in a few. These and other studies of prophylactic granulocyte transfusion failed to show a positive effect on the rate or duration of remission or survival of acute leukemic patients.

There are many potential disadvantages to prophylactic granulocyte transfusion including: increased sensitization to WBC antigens rendering future transfusions more difficult; graft-versus-host disease; and transmission of viral diseases, especially cytomegalovirus (CMV). In their retrospective analysis of a large number of allogeneic bone marrow transplant recipients, Hersman et al. (15) have shown that patients receiving prophylactic granulocyte transfusions have an increased chance of excreting CMV in their urine. More important, CMV seronegative patients receiving transfused cells from seropositive donors have a significantly high incidence of CMV interstitial pneumonitis compared to seronegative transplant patients not given prophylactic granulocytes. The risk of CMV interstitial pneumonia was lower in seronegative patients transfused from comparable seronegative donors (15). Another disadvantage of prophylactic granulocyte transfusion is lethal pulmonary reactions associated with the combined use of Amphotericin B and granulocyte transfusions (16). Acute respiratory deterioration occurred in 64% of the patients when Amphotericin B was given at some time during the course of granulocyte transfusion compared to 6% when Amphotericin B was given alone. These patients had begun taking amphotericin B at or after the initiation of granulocyte transfusions, and in all but one of these patients the respiratory deterioration began during the first four days of therapy, when amphotericin B reactions are typically most severe. Most severe respiratory symptoms were seen during or shortly after a granulocyte transfusion. Our conclusion at this time is that there is no role for prophylactic granulocyte transfusions.

There are two major factors which are often ignored in clinical situations: granulocyte dose and histocompatibility factors. The importance of the dose-response relationship has been described in many clinical and experimental studies (8,17-19). Normal granulocyte turnover is 10^{10} cells/day, and increases two- to four-fold during infectious stress. The average granulocyte yield from a single session of leukapheresis (without steroid premedication of the donor) is 5-10 x 10^9 cells which is less than 10% of normal granulocyte turnover. Although improvement of infection is seen after using this dose, many investigators believe that the few negative studies of both therapeutic and prophylactic granulocyte transfusion trials may be due to the low dose of granulocytes.

One source of larger numbers of granulocytes for transfusion is the population of patients with chronic myelocytic leukemia (CML) due to their high circulating leukocyte count. Although used extensively in the developmental stages of granulocyte transfusion (17), normal donors are now used in most centers. In an attempt to maximize granulocyte dose, Schiffer et al. (20) have again begun to utilize donors with CML in the supportive care of seriously infected patients. Fourteen patients with acute leukemia received CML leukocyte transfusions for the treatment of 16 infectious episodes. Sustained granulocyte count increments with PMN greater than 500/cu. mm. following the last CML transfusion were seen in 7 of 10 evaluable transfusion episodes. Two patients had engraftment demonstrated by the presence of the Ph^1 and sex chromosomes. Resolution of signs and symptoms of infection was seen in 6 patients and seemed to correlate with the persistence of granulocytes after transfusion.

A relationship between donor and recipient histocompatibility and post transfusion granulocyte recovery has also been demonstrated (21). Using an identical twin as the donor for granulocyte transfusions, the granulocyte increment 1 hour post transfusion was 42%. Using an HLA and ABO compatible donor the granulocyte increment was 50%; this decreased to 5% for patients who received HLA compatible but ABO incompatible donor granulocytes (21). A recent study using the radioisotope indium-111 oxine-labelled granulocytes demonstrated a lack of granulocyte migration to sites of infection for alloimmunized patients identified clinically by refractoriness to platelet transfusion along with a history of prior transfusion reactions (22). While the therapeutic advantage of donor/recipient histocompatibility is evident, it is not practical to match all antigens due to the presence of both HLA antigens and granulocyte specific antigens on the surface of neutrophils. In the hope that granulocyte-specific antigens are more likely to be identical in the family setting (23), we therefore recommend using compatible platelet donors as granulocyte donors with a preference for family members.

3. PLATELET TRANSFUSION

As reported by Howard and Perkins (24), seventy percent of patients with various hematological diseases requiring repeated platelet transfusions eventually become refractory to later transfusions. The number of platelet concentrates or transfusion episodes required to induce antibodies varies greatly among individual patients. Dutcher et al. (25) studied 114 patients with acute nonlymphocytic leukemia and reported that: 1) 58% of patients had no lymphocytotoxic antibody from the time of admission to 6-8 weeks post-chemotherapy; 2) 30% of those who had lymphocytotoxic antibody on admission became alloimmunized during the induction period; and 3) the remaining 12% demonstrated either alloimmunization on admission or anamnestic antibody response within 1 week of transfusion. Of the patients who showed no antibody during initial therapy (58%), 92% will continue to test negative. This data allows prospective identification of a group of patients who can receive more intensive maintenance chemotherapy with relative safety since they can be easily supported with random donor platelets. Only 40% of newly diagnosed ANLL patients will require HLA matched platelet transfusions early in the course of the therapy, although the use of single donor platelets from the beginning of therapy has become common in many blood centers. Considering the donor risk, increased expense, and the relatively small population of patients to be benefited, the use of single donor platelets for patients with leukemia should be limited to alloimmunized patients except in investigational settings.

In general, spontaneous bleeding from thrombocytopenia does not occur until circulating platelets drop below 20,000/cu. mm. (26). Some patients may remain stable despite lower platelet counts (less than 10,000/cu. mm.) while others may develop spontaneous bleeding at counts of 40-50,000/cu. mm. There are two general approaches to platelet therapy: 1) to transfuse when there is clinical evidence of bleeding or 2) to transfuse as prophylaxis against bleeding when platelets are below 20,000/cu. mm. Careful clinical trials have shown that prophylactic platelet transfusions can reduce the incidence of bleeding and its associated morbidity compared to transfusions given only after bleeding starts (27,28). The rate of decrease in platelet numbers as well as other factors responsible for platelet consumption (infection, bleeding) should be considered in determining at what platelet level replacement therapy should be initiated. The most reliable and practical tests to evaluate platelet transfusion response is the measurement of platelet increment after transfusion. Post-transfusion platelet counts are measured at 1 hour and 24 hours after transfusion. The 1-hour count indicates platelet recovery and the 24-hour count shows the survival of transfused platelets. In order to compare between patients of different sizes and weights, receiving different amounts of platelets, additional calculations must be made. Grumet and Yankee (29) used the following formula for the corrected increment.

$$\text{Corrected Increment} = \frac{\text{Observed increment x BSA}}{\text{No. of units transfused}}$$

BSA represents the body surface in M^2. A compatible response has been estimated as being an increment of more than 7500/cu. mm. at 1 hour and greater than 4500/cu. mm. at 24 hours.

Aster (30) developed another method to calculate the percentage recovery (or increment) with the formula:

$$\text{\% Recovery} = \frac{\text{Observed increment x blood volume x 100\%}}{\text{No. of platelets transfused x 0.67}}$$

The correction factor of 0.67 accounts for obligatory splenic pooling of one-third of transfused platelets and is omitted if the recipient is splenectomized (30).

Failure to achieve a significant platelet transfusion response may occur in many clinical conditions (intracorporeal factors) which affect platelet recovery or survival: sepsis, disseminated intravascular coagulation, bleeding, splenomegaly, or exposure to certain drugs leading to immune mediated platelet destruction. Extracorporeal factors which may compromise platelet transfusion recovery include method of collection, type of anticoagulant, pH of the preparation, temperature and duration of storage, donor antiplatelet medication, and dose of platelets. Platelet concentrates containing incompatible leukocytes may also be less effective in recipients who have circulating leukoagglutinins. These causes of refractoriness must be ruled out before one can assume that platelets matched for the appropriate antigens will be more effective. If all of the above causes of refractoriness can be ruled out, it is likely that a poor platelet increment is the result of alloimmunization and attempts to provide HLA compatible platelets should be initiated.

Refractoriness is defined as failure on at least two occasions to achieve a significant platelet increment after a reasonable dose of platelets. The latent period for alloimmunization is usually shorter in patients with a history of blood transfusions or multiple pregnancies. Many studies have shown that HLA antibodies play a major role in the refractory state. The antigens of the HLA-A and B locus are the most immunogenic of the various antigens expressed on the platelet surface. Other non-HLA antigens appear to be less important but may also provoke refractoriness in some patients. ABO and HLA-C antigens are expressed in lower quantitites on platelet membrane, thus have little influence on alloimmunization. HLA-D, DR, and Rhesus antigens are believed to be absent from platelets. Because of the polymorphism of the HLA system, long-term transfusion support using "perfectly matched" HLA-A and HLA-B donors is not practical in most circumstances. Lohrmann et al. (31) demonstrated that Grade B matched platelets (i.e., the donor and recipient sharing two or three HLA antigens, the donor having no HLA antigen in excess of the recipient and the donor's HLA type showing one or two blanks) were as effective as fully compatible (grade A) platelets. Experimental evidence has suggested that cross-reactive antigens have relatively low immunogenicity in transplant or transfusion recipients. Duquesnoy et al. (32) have evaluated the effectiveness of platelets selectively mismatched for cross-reactive HLA antigens in alloimmunized thrombocytopenic patients and found that the yield from such platelets is only slightly less than that with a "perfect" match. Using donor selection criteria which include cross-reactive HLA antigens, one can expand the donor pool size by tenfold and thus improve the practicality of HLA-compatible platelet tranfusion. Computer programs have been developed to facilitate the search for a compatible donor by making use of cross-reactive antigens.

In spite of availability of HLA matched platelets, 20% of refractory patients fail to respond to such transfusions due to: 1) the presence of antibodies to non-HLA antigens; 2) the innocent bystander destruction of platelet due to incompatible granulocytes present in platelet concentrates; 3) the presence of antibodies against Bw4/Bw6 antigen system. The Bw4/Bw6 antigen system is a biallelic system of HLA antigens closely related to HLA-B that has been detected on lymphocytes and platelets by serologic methods. HLA-B antigens that are cross-reactive sometimes differ in their Bw4/Bw6 specificities. When alloimmunized thrombocytopenic patients were transfused with Bw4/Bw6 compatible platelets 8 of 21 patients (38%) experienced a satisfactory platelet increment at 1 and 24 hours post transfusion while failing to respond to Bw4/Bw6-incompatible transfusions (33).

In order to delay alloimmunization in patients with acute leukemia undergoing induction chemotherapy, Swiss investigators have reported (34) the results of a randomized study using random single-donor vs. multiple-donor platelet transfusion. Of the 54 patients entered onto the study, the frequency of alloantibody formation, time periods and numbers of transfusion to acquire refractoriness was reduced in patients randomized to receive single-donor platelet transfusions. Furthermore, the increments decreased from the first to the last transfusion in patients receiving multiple-donor platelets, compared to the group receiving single-donor platelets who maintained essentially the same level of increments throughout the study period. The benefit of this transfusion policy was particularly evident in patients with previous pregnancies. More data will be needed to address this important issue because of the expense and limited apheresis donors; routine use of single-donor platelet transfusion is not justified.

Recent advances in cryobiology have encouraged the development of an autologous frozen platelet transfusion program at the University of Maryland Cancer Center, representing about 15% of the total transfusions administered to patients with leukemia at that Center. Their data show that frozen platelets were effective in stopping clinical bleeding with significant rise in post-transfusion increments (35). If this method can be widely adapted by other centers, autologous frozen platelets will be the best choice for the selective group of patients who fail to respond to HLA matched platelets.

ACKNOWLEDGEMENT

The authors wish to thank Father Joe Mahoney for his help with this manuscript.

REFERENCES

1. Goldfinger D: Prevention of transfusion reaction by the use of saline washed packed red cells. Prog. in Clin. Bio. Research 65:59-67, 1981.
2. Van Zant G, Goldwasser E, Pech N: Competition between erythropoietin and colony-stimulating factor for target cells in mouse marrow. Blood 53:946-965, 1979.
3. Hahn CM, Schimff SC, Fortner CL et al: Infection in acute leukemia patients receiving oral nonabsorbable antibiotics. Antimicrob. Agents Chemother. 13:958-964, 1978.
4. Love LH, Schimff SC, Schiffer CA et al: Improved prognosis for granulocytic patients with gram-negative bacteremia. Amer. J. Med. 68:643-648, 1980.

5. EORTC International Antimicrobial Therapy Project Group: Three antibiotic regimens in the treatment of infection in febrile granulocytopenic patients with cancer. J. Infect. Dis. 137:14-29, 1978.
6. Klastersky J: Combinations of antibiotics for therapy of severe infections in cancer patients. Eur. J. Cancer 14: 3-13, 1979.
7. Bodey GP, Buckley M, Sathe US, Freireich EJ: Quantitative relationships between circulating leukocytes and infection in patients with acute leukemia. Ann. Int. Med. 64:328-340, 1966.
8. Appelbaum FR, Bowles CA, Makuch RW et al: Granulocyte transfusion therapy of experimental pseudomonas septicemia: Study of cell dose and collection technique. Blood 52:323-331, 1978.
9. Herzig RH, Herzig GP, Graw RG, Jr et al: Successful granulocyte transfusion therapy for gram-negative septicemia. NEJM 296:701-705, 1977.
10. Winston DJ, Ho WG, Gale RP: Therapeutic granulocyte transfusion for documented infections. Ann. Int. Med. 97:509-515, 1982.
11. Love LJ, Schimpff SC, Schiffer CA, Wierhik PH: Improved prognosis for granulocytopenic patients with gram negative septicemia. Amer. J. Med. 68:643-648, 1980.
12. Higby DJ, Burnett D: Granulocyte transfusion: Current status. Blood 55:2-8, 1980.
13. Strauss RG, Connett JE, Gale RP et al: A controlled trial of prophylactic granulocyte transfusions during initial induction chemotherapy for acute myelogenous leukemia. NEJM 305:597-603, 1981.
14. Clift RA, Sanders JE, Thomas ED: Granulocyte transfusions for the prevention of infection in patients receiving bone marrow transplants. NEJM 298:1052-1057, 1978.
15. Hersman J, Meyers JD, Thomas ED, Buckner CD: The effect of granulocyte transfusion on the incidence of cytomegalovirus infection after allogeneic marrow transplantation. Ann. Int. Med. 96:149-150, 1982.
16. Wright DG, Robichand KJ, Pizzo P, Deisseroth AB: Lethal pulmonary reactions associated with combined use of amphotericin B and leukocyte transfusion. NEJM 304: 1184-1189, 1981.
17. Freireich EJ, Levin RH, Whang J et al: The function and fate of transfused leukocytes from donors with chronic myelocytic leukemia in leukopenic recipients. Ann. NY Acad. Sci. 113:1081-1089, 1964.
18. Higby DJ, Freeman A, Henderson ES et al: Granulocyte transfusion in children using filter collected cells. Cancer 38:1407-1413, 1976.
19. Epstein RB, Chow HS: An analysis of quantitative relationships of granulocyte transfusion therapy in canines. Transfusion 21:360-362, 1981.

20. Schiffer CA, Aisner J, Dutcher JP, Wiernik PH: Sustained post-transfusion granulocyte count increments following transfusion of leukocytes obtained from donors with chronic myelogenous leukemia. Amer. J. Hematol. 14:65-74, 1983.
21. Herzig GP, Graw RG: Granulocyte transfusion for bacterial infections. In: Progress in Hematology, Vol. XII, 1981, pp. 207-228.
22. Dutcher JP, Schiffer CA, Johnson GS et al: Alloimmunization prevents the migration of transfused indium-111-labeled granulocytes to sites of infection. Blood 62: 354-360, 1983.
23. Schiffer, CA: Granulocyte transfusion therapy. Cancer Treat. Rep. 67:113-119, 1983.
24. Howard JE, Perkins HA: The natural history of alloimmunization to platelets. Transfusion 18:496-503, 1978.
25. Dutcher JP, Schiffer CA, Aisner J, Wiernik PH: Longterm follow up of patients with acute leukemia receiving platelet transfusions: Identification of a large group of patients who do not become alloimmunized. Blood 58:1007-1011, 1981.
26. Gaydos L, Freireich EJ, Mantel N: Orientation relation between platelet count and hemorrhage in patients with acute leukemia. NEJM 266:905-909, 1962.
27. Higby DJ, Cohen E, Holland JF, Sinks L: The prophylactic treatment of thrombocytopenic leukemic patients with platelets: A double blind study. Transfusion 14:440-446, 1974.
28. Murphy S, Koch PA, Evans AE: Randomized trial of prophylactic vs. therapeutic platelet transfusion in childhood acute leukemia. Clin. Res. 24:379a, 1976.
29. Grumet FC, Yankee RA: Long term platelet support of patients with aplastic anemia: Effect of splenectomy and steroid therapy. Ann. Int. Med. 73:1-7, 1970.
30. Aster RH: Pooling of platelets in the spleen: Role in the pathogenesis of "hypersplenic" thrombocytopenia. J. Clin. Inv. 45:645-657, 1966.
31. Lohrmann HP, Bull MI, Decter JA et al: Platelet transfusions from HLA compatible unrelated donors to alloimmunized patients. Ann. Int. Med. 80:9-14, 1974.
32. Duquensnoy RJ, Filip DJ, Rodey GE et al: Successful transfusion of platelet "mismatched" for HLA antigens to alloimmunized thrombocytopenic patients. Amer. J. Hematol. 2:219-226, 1977.
33. McElligott MC, Menitove JE, Duquesnoy RJ et al: Effect of HLA Bw4/Bw6 compatibility on platelet transfusion response of refractory thrombocytopenic patients. Blood 59:971-975, 1982.
34. Gmur J, Von Felten A, Osterwalder B et al: Delayed alloimmunization using random single donor platelet transfusions: A prospective study in thrombocytopenic patients with acute leukemia. Blood 62:473-479, 1983.

35. Schiffer CA, Aisner J, Dutcher JP: Platelet cryopreservation using dimethyl sulfoxide. Ann. N.Y. Acad. Sci. 411:161-169, 1983.

17

LEUKEMIA: HEMORRHAGIC AND THROMBOTIC COMPLICATIONS

Dr. John Penner

Hemorrhagic and thrombotic problems occur commonly in the course of the leukemias and vary in relation to the form of the leukemia and programs of management. In most instances, supporting measures in the form of platelet concentrates or anticoagulants have been effective in controlling such manifestations, at least for short periods. These complications in relation to their underlying process and its expression are listed in Table 1. Note that disseminated intravascular coagulation presents itself in relation to thrombosis as well as hemorrhage.

Table 1. Leukemia: Complications

Hemorrhage	Thrombosis
Thrombocytopenia	Thrombocytosis
Thrombocytopathy	Leukocytosis
Vitamin K Deficiency	Antithrombin III Deficiency
Consumption Coagulopathy	Intravascular Coagulation

1. HEMORRHAGIC COMPLICATIONS

1.1 Thrombocytopenia

The majority of bleeding problems associated with leukemia are due to a lack of adequate numbers of platelets. When seen initially, thrombocytopenia usually is a result of megakaryocyte displacement by the overgrowth of leukemic cells in the marrow.

Eventually with treatment, megakaryocyte damage by chemotherapeutic agents becomes the major contributor to platelet depletion. Less common forms of thrombocytopenia also can occur as a result of platelet destruction by drug action or immune mechanisms, or simply through increased utilization as seen in the consumption coagulopathies.

Platelet production can be assessed easily by examining a marrow aspirate or biopsy. The absence of megakaryocytes either in the presence of extensive leukemic cell infiltration, or in a hypoplastic marrow following chemotherapy, identifies disorders of production. If megakaryocytes persist, however, destruction or utilization must be considered. Heparin, antibiotics, several diuretics, and many other drugs can damage platelets directly or induce an immune reaction, producing thrombocytopenia without megakaryocytopenia. Discontinuing a potentially offensive drug or eliminating a Heparin flush allows rapid recovery of platelets within a period of 3 to 4 days and provides the best means of diagnosis. In some instances, addition of the drug and patient plasma to normal platelets can produce a diagnostic clumping reaction.

Isoimmune problems are not so easily identified or managed. Platelet typing is offered in some institutions (adding the patient's plasma to platelets obtained from normal donors) and may permit recognition of a platelet isoantibody. Approximately 2% of the population lack a common antigen PLa_1 and can develop antibodies after exposure to PLa_1 containing platelets (1). The antibodies will destroy infused as well as the patient's own platelets. This is a rare occurrence however, while destruction of transfused platelets in multi-transfused patients by antibodies to the human lymphocyte antigens (HLA) is a much more frequent problem (2). The patients response to HLA matched platelets assessed at one hour after injection will determine the significance of this source of immune damage.

Platelet comsumption or utilization also must be considered, particularly in septic patients or in those who develop rapid and extensive cell lysis. A broader evaluation of the clotting mechanism; measurement of fibrinogen, Antithrombin III and fibrin degradation products can be definitive.

Unfortunately, it is not always possible to identify the etiology of thrombocytopenia, inasmuch as leukemic disorders often present, not only with decreased platelet production as a result of megakaryocytopenia, but also with increased utilization related to sepsis, and elements of immune destruction as well, especially of transfused platelets.

1.2 Management

Management of thrombocytopenia in leukemic patients requires good clinical judgement and some knowledge of the platelet requirements for hemostasis. Normal functioning platelets circulating at a level of 10,000/mm^3 generally are sufficient to provide hemostasis and prevent spontaneous bleeding. Studies undertaken by Shihadeh and Penner (3), Figures 1, 2, evaluated thrombocytopenic patients in relation to bleeding manifestations on a scale of 0 to 4. Severe bleeding requiring platelet transfusions was designated as 4, with more moderate bleeding phenomena scaled from 0 to 3. As seen in Figure 1, serious bleeding was seldom encountered with platelet counts of greater than 10,000, while little if any bleeding was observed with counts of greater than 50,000/mm^3. Recognizing the fact that platelet function is more important than platelet numbers, the same patients were examined with respect to the Ivy bleeding time. A strong correlation between bleeding time and platelet count existed. As seen in Figure 2, the bleeding time and bleeding manifestations also correlated well. Serious bleeding was seldom encountered unless the bleeding time was greater than 15 minutes. Notice in both Figures, a group of patients were seen who have less than 10,000 platelets with bleeding times greater than 15 minutes and no significant bleeding problem. This group of patients represented many younger individuals whose vascular integrity perhaps was better. Other factors which should be considered are the steroid levels (adrenal corticoids and androgens will reduce capillary fragility) and the duration of the patient's thrombocytopenia. Spontaneous bleeding is more apt to occur in those individuals whose platelet counts have been persistently below 10,000/mm^3 for a number of days. From the clinical standpoint, the appearance of mucosal hemorrhage is of greatest significance and warrants therapeutic intervention. Petechiae, particularly over the lower extremities, are not infrequent findings in thrombocytopenic patients, and unless a shower of fresh lesions are seen, should not necessarily give cause for alarm.

Thus, the risk factors that should be assessed before initiating therapy with platelet concentrates are clinical signs of bleeding, particularly from the mucosa; the number of platelets circulating; the bleeding time; the age of the patient; and the duration of thrombocytopenia.

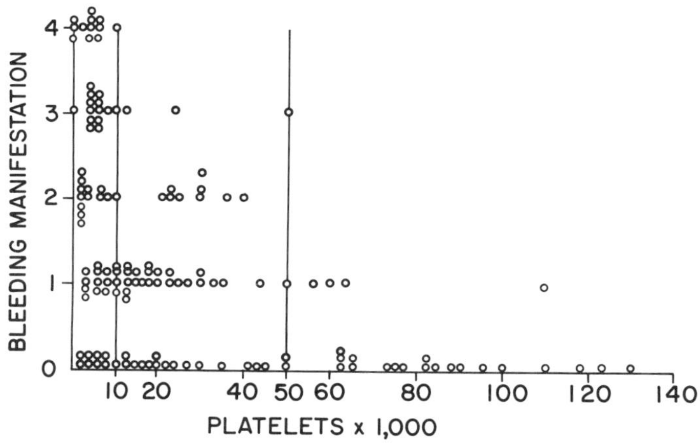

Figure 1. Thrombocytopenia: Bleeding in relation to platelet count.

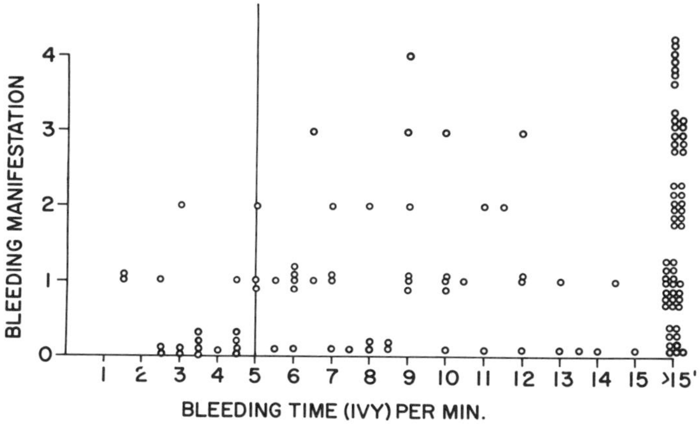

Figure 2. Thrombocytopenia: Bleeding in relation to bleeding time (Ivy).

1.3 Platelet concentrates

As prepared by American Red Cross and Community Blood Banks, concentrates are required to contain 5 x 10^{10} platelets/bag, and can be irradiated to eliminate lymphocytes with their risk of a possible graft vs. host reaction. Ordinarily, 1 to 2 bags/ 10 Kg body weight are administered, depending on the presence of active bleeding or the seriousness of the bleeding risk. Initial treatment usually consists of platelets from random donors, although single unit donor platelets may be less prone to sensitize the patient. Continued "random" platelet transfusions eventually induce antibody formation (approximately 60% of multi-transfused patients) with resulting rapid loss of platelets due to agglutination and a decrease in the duration of benefit. Platelet counts obtained 1 hour post infusion provide a means of evaluating such immune reactions. If the patient fails to obtain a significant increase at 1 hour, HLA

Typed Platelets should be considered, and are available at many Blood Banking Centers. A 4 antigen match often can be provided with subsequent improvement in the 1 hour platelet recovery. In some patients, immune reactions to HLA Matched Platelets results in agglutination and rapid disappearance. Even in these situations, administration of platelets may be of value for short periods of time. Certainly patients who are bleeding as a result of thrombocytopenia should not have platelets withheld simply because it has not been possible to increase the circulating level. Other supportive measures include the use of steroids, which for short periods reduce capillary fragility, and Epsilon Amino Caproic Acid (Amicar), an anti-fibrinolytic agent which inhibits the plasminogen activator and helps to maintain the integrity of the hemostatic clot.

1.4 Thrombocytopathia

Platelet bleeding disorders also must be considered with respect to platelet dysfunction. Many of the antibiotics that are employed to manage infectious complications (Table 2), penicillins and the cephalosporins, inhibit platelet aggregation and platelet release, thus contributing to bleeding tendencies (4). Severity of the problem can be judged on the basis of the bleeding time and can be demonstrated by a platelet aggregation study in which the patient's platelet rich plasma fails to respond to aggregating agents, ADP and Epinephrine. The dysfunction may be severe enough to require alteration in the antibiotic program. Note the uremia also induces a qualitative platelet defect and can be alleviated by improvement in the uremic state through dialysis or, perhaps as recently described, with the use of a new pitressin analogue, DDAVP, which increases the circulating von Willebrand Factor (5). Platelet concentrate administration can improve these disorders temporarily, however, the effectiveness of the transfused platelets disappears rapidly.

Table 2. Antibiotics and Platelet Dysfunction

Penicillins	Cephalosporins
Penicillin G	Cefamandole*
Carbenicillin	Cefmetazole
Ticarcillin	Cefmanoxamine
Ampicillin	Moxalactam*
	Cefaperazone*

* Also produce decrease in functional activity Vitamin K dependent clotting factors.

1.5 Plasma coagulation factors

Deficiency of the Vitamin K dependent factors has become a recognized problem in the leukemic patient only recently. The aggressive approach to therapy presently employed often requires patients to be maintained on intravenous feedings which lack Vitamin K, while the addition of broad spectrum antibiotics also reduces bacterial production of Vitamin K in the large bowl. This lack of Vitamin compromises the carboxylation of glutamic acid residues on Prothrombin Factors VII, IX and X, preventing these proteases from combining with calcium on phospholipid surfaces, an interaction required for thrombin formation. Most recently, the cephalosporin antibiotics and third generation penicillins have been found to interrupt the carboxylation process in a manner similar to the oral anticoagulant, Warfarin, resulting in a prolongation of the Prothrombin Time and the Partial Thromboplastin Time (6). Bleeding manifestations under these conditions of aggressive therapy have been observed. Prolonged clotting times in the presence of normal levels of fibrinogen provide a relatively simple means of identifying this problem. Administration of Vitamin K_1 (Mephyton), 10 mg. orally or intravenously, produces a significant improvement in laboratory values within a 12 to 24 hour period. Needless to say, active bleeding should be managed by replacement of factors through use of plasma, 10 ml/Kg while awaiting the expected improvement from Vitamin K.

As previously described, the antibiotic problem also manifests itself by inducing platelet dysfunction. The combination of defects in both plasma clotting factors and platelets often results in serious bleeding which can be avoided by altering the antibiotic program.

1.6 Consumption coagulopathies

Intravascular coagulation creates hemorrhagic as well as thrombotic problems, and will be described in more detail under the section of Thrombosis. With respect to the associated bleeding manifestations, support in the form of platelet concentrates provides the best means of management. Such concentrates contain many of the clotting factors needed to correct the hemostatic disorder; for example, platelets contain Factor V and fibrinogen, and in addition, considerable quantities of Factor VIII and Factor V are present in the surrounding plasma envelope. Most platelet concentrates now consist of a 50 ml. volume of relatively fresh plasma, and thus 10 to 12 concentrates provide significant amounts of many of the needed clotting factors as well as platelets. The Prothrombin Time and Partial Thromboplastin Time can be monitored to determine the need for additional plasma. Ordinarily, 10 mg/Kg of fresh frozen plasma is sufficient to improve hemostasis in these conditions if platelet concentrates have not been effective. Lastly, when fibrinogen levels are markedly reduced, Cryoprecipitate or Cryo Factor VIII is available in most regions of the country, and contain approximately 200 mg. of fibrinogen in addition to 100 units of Factor VIII/10 ml. bag. Ten bags of Cryoprecipitate provide a very effective means of replacing fibrinogen and Factor VIII, and perhaps provide some additional benefit from their content of Fibronectin and the von Willebrand Factor.

1.7 Treatment

In all instances, correction of hemostatic complications can best be achieved by rapid infusion of the blood byproducts, be it platelets or fresh frozen plasma, or Cryoprecipitate. Ordinarily infusion time should be limited to 30 minutes unless the patients cardiac status does not permit a rapid increase in blood volume. Thus 10 to 12 platelet concentrates can be infused within a half hour. Fresh frozen plasma, 10 units/Kg may require a somewhat longer period. For maximum benefit, however, the rapid increase in circulating clotting factors is necessary to provide an effective hemostatic level.

2. THROMBOTIC COMPLICATIONS

Thrombosis, surprisingly, is not uncommon in leukemic disorders and is most frequently found in situations where cell counts are very high, antithrombin levels are depressed, or sepsis and/or tissue destruction have created conditions which accelerate coagulation.

2.1 Leukocytosis and thrombocytosis

Chronic granulocytic leukemia, for example, often exhibits marked thrombocytosis as do related disorders - thrombocythemia and polycythemia. In these situations, the excessive numbers of platelets, sometimes exceeding 4,000,000, may produce hemorrhagic manifestations, perhaps as a result of the qualitative platelet dysfunction as well as thrombotic complications. Leukocytosis in these same disorders, and in acute forms of myeloid leukemia also can create similar problems, particularly when the white cell hematocrit or buffy layer is increased to levels of 20 volumes % or more. These granulocytic cells often appear to stick together in clumps and occlude small vessels of the brain and kidney producing rapid and irreversible damage.

In the past, management of these conditions has depended entirely upon use of rapidly effective chemotherapeutic agents such as Hydroxyurea in chronic granulocytic leukemia, Methotrexate and Cytosine Arabinoside in acute leukemia. Often, however, a catastrophe occurs before the response to the chemotherapy, or develops as a result of the accelerated coagulation induced by chemotherapies rapid cell lysis and a release of tissue substances (thromboplastin). Leukopheresis or thrombocytopheresis offers an immediate effective approach to management. A 3 to 4 liter removal of platelet and leukocyte rich plasma from the patient daily for 2 to 3 days will provide a rapid reduction in cell count and reduce the risk of thrombotic events. Such procedures should be reserved for patients with platelet counts of >2,000,000/mm^3 or leukocyte counts (granulocytes) >200,000, or those with manifestations of thrombosis.

2.2 Antithrombin deficiency

L-Asparaginase, one of the chemotherapeutic agents commonly employed for treatment of acute lymphocytic leukemia, has the capacity to increase the risk of thrombosis by reducing Antithrombin III, the major protease inhibitor in the circulation. In a recent study using a standard induction regimen for acute leukemia, reduction not only of Antithrombin III, but plasminogen and fibrinogen were observed while platelet aggregation was noted to be increased as was Factor V and VIII (7). Thus, an increased risk for thrombotic events may develop and should be considered when using this agent alone or in combination. Antithrombin III concentrate, which soon may be approved for use in this country, plasma and/or Heparin offer a means of reducing this risk particularly in patients who are inactive and maintained at bed rest.

2.3 Intravascular coagulation

Consumption coagulopathies have been alluded to with respect to bleeding manifestations as well as its relation to thrombosis. The basis of this risk in the leukemic patient resides in both the extrinsic and intrinsic aspects of the coagulation mechanism. Gram negative sepsis creates endotoxin damage to the endothelium and rapid utilization of platelets on the damaged surfaces with release of phospholipids and thromboxane. The latter produces platelet aggregation and vasoconstriction while the former initiates thrombin formation with resulting fibrin deposition along the walls of the larger arteries. Where vasoconstriction or vascular irregularity decreases the blood flow, an occlusive thrombus may develop.

Thromboplastin release from leukocytes or necrotic tissue following chemotherapy rapidly activates the extrinsic system with formation of the protease Factor Xa, and finally large amounts of thrombin. This action again results in fibrin formation along vessel walls or in an occlusive thrombus. One form of leukemia, the progranulocytic variety, is particularly prone to this development. The large numbers of progranulocytes present in the marrow and blood in this condition, apparently are able to activate the clotting mechanism through the release of thromboplastin-like substances. In this situation more than others, hypofibrinogenemia is common and represents the major manifestation of the intravascular coagulation syndrome. Some activation of the fibrinolytic system also appears with destruction of fibrinogen and fibrin by plasmin (8).

In all instances, diagnosis depends upon assays that can identify a decrease in factors consumed when blood clots (Table 3). In this process, platelets decrease in the circulation as they are aggregated by thrombin, thromboxane, epinephrin or adenosine diphosphate; prothrombin is converted to thrombin; fibrinogen to fibrin; and Factor V and Factor VIII are destroyed by thrombin, perhaps through the activation of Protein C. Antithrombin III also is depleted as it binds with the proteases and is removed from the circulation. Fibrin degradation products (FdP) build up as fibrin monomer is formed by thrombin's action, and degradation of fibrinogen and fibrin results from activation of plasminogen. Platelet and fibrinogen values are most easily followed, however, and are the basis of diagnosis. Many of our leukemic patients are thrombocytopenic to begin with, however, and the fibrinogen level may be the only useful value. Prothrombin Time and Partial Thromboplastin Time will become prolonged as a result of the decreased Factor V, Factor VIII and fibrinogen, while measurement of Antithrombin III and the fibrin degradation products may provide additional support for the diagnosis.

Table 3. Intravascular Coagulation

Clotting Factors			Related Laboratory Procedures	
Platelets	-Dec	...	Platelet Count	-Dec
Prothrombin	-Dec	...	P.T. and A.P.T.T.	-Inc
Factor V and VIII	-Dec	...	P.T. and A.P.T.T.	-Inc
Fibrinogen	-Dec	...	Fibrinogen P.T. and A.P.T.T.	-Dec -Inc
Antithrombin III	-Dec	...	AT III	-Dec
Fibrin Degradation Products	-Inc	...	Latex Aggregation (T-W) Protamine Sulfate Flocculation	-Inc -Pos

Certain characteristics of intravascular coagulation can be employed to identify the etiology of this disorder. Release of endotoxin from gram negative organisms initially produces a thrombocytopenia followed by activation of plasma clotting factors leading to a late appearing depletion of fibrinogen. Note that many infections may produce a secondary rise in fibrinogen and, therefore, fibrinogen levels may appear normal or elevated initially and gradually decline over a period of hours to days. Thromboplastin release associated with progranulocytic leukemia or with a rapid destruction of leukocytes may produce a much more rapid decline in fibrinogen since activation of the clotting factors occurs directly. Platelets tend to fall much later under these circumstances.

The therapeutic approach in this situation with respect to hemorrhage has been mentioned, replacement of platelets generally will control bleeding. Use of Cryoprecipitate and fresh frozen plasma also may be beneficial. Thrombotic complications, however, require a somewhat different approach. Anticoagulant therapy in the form of Heparin should be considered if thrombosis and hemorrhagic infarction present a problem. In those patients who develop a hypotensive episode, for example, renal blood flow is reduced and microthrombi appear in the kidney, leading to renal necrosis. Hemorrhagic infarction of the skin and other organs, as seen in Purpura Fulminans, also may indicate intravascular thrombus formation and the necessity for using Heparin. Ordinarily, low dose Heparin, 5,000 units subcutaneously at 8 hour intervals, can be initiated to control the process. If thrombosis appears extensive, a more therapeutic regimen can be offered with a dose of 100 units/Kg by constant infusion every 6 or 8 hours. Heparin should not be considered if bleeding is present, or if there are signs of central nervous system hemorrhage. Control of bleeding by infusion of platelet concentrates should be established before Heparin therapy is initiated. Antithrombin III concentrates, when available, also may prove to be effective, alone or with Heparin. If the Antithrombin III levels are low, less than 50%, use of fresh frozen plasma, 10 ml/Kg will increase the circulating level and enhance the effects of Heparin.

2.4 Summary

Hemorrhagic and thrombotic manifestations of leukemias are difficult to evaluate, inasmuch as one of the major elements in hemostasis, the platelets, often are decreased as a result of the leukemic process itself. Determining the basis of the thrombocytopenia, be it utilization or immune destruction, frequently is difficult, and certainly in the diagnosis of intravascular coagulation, it is often necessary to rely on the assessment of other clotting factors. Treatment for the most part is readily available. Hemostatic problems generally can be managed with platelet concentrates, and only when complex immune problems result in rapid destruction of infused platelets are we faced with a difficult situation. Even in these instances, the short-lived platelets may be effective, perhaps with plasmapheresis to reduce the level of damaging antibodies. Steroids and the fibrinolytic activator inhibitor EACA also may provide some additional support. Our most obstinate problem at the moment remains that of antibiotic induced damage to platelet function. It may not be possible to offer other alternatives without reducing the effectiveness of our treatment for infection. In some cases, it may be necessary to provide continued platelet support while such agents are being used, even though the patient's own platelets were adequate prior to the use of antibiotics. Appropriate administration of Vitamin K always should be considered during antibiotic therapy, and careful laboratory monitoring of hemostasis is a necessity. Cryoprecipitates and fresh frozen plasma with their available plasma clotting factors can provide supplemental support for control of hemostasis in the consumption coagulopathies. In situations where thrombotic problems have arisen, the use of anticoagulants, Heparin and Antithrombin III, may be of value, while leuko and thrombocytopheresis provide opportunities for reducing immediate risks imposed by elevated circulating levels of granulocytes and platelets.

REFERENCES

1. Shulman NR, et al: Immunoreactions involving platelets vs. post transfusion purpura due to a complement fixing antibody against genetically controlled platelet antigen. J. Clin. Invest. 40:1597-1603, 1961.

2. Schlicter JS: Controversies in platelet transfusion therapy. Ann. Rev. Med. 31:509, 1980.
3. Shihadeh M, Penner JA: Unpublished data.
4. Brown CH, Natelson EA, Bradshaw MW, et al: The hemostatic defect produced by carbenacillin. N. Eng. J. Med. 291: 265-270, 1974.
5. Mannucci PM, Remuzzi G, et al: Deamino-8-d-arginine vasopressin shortens bleeding time in uremia. N. Eng. J. Med. 308:8-12, 1983.
6. Hooper CA, Haney BB, Stone AH: Gastrointestinal bleeding due to vitamin K deficiency in patients on parenteral cefamandol. Lancet 1:39-40, 1980.
7. Pui C, Jackson CW, Chesney C, et al: Change in platelet function and coagulation in leukemic children treated with L-asparaginase, prednisone, vincristine. J. Clin. Onc. 1:380-385, 1983.
8. Didisheim P, et al: Acute promyelocytic leukemia with fibrinogen and factor V deficiencies. Blood 23:717, 1964.